A Diet You Can Live With

Turning the quest for vitamins, proteins, antioxidants, phytochemicals, prebiotics, fibers and more, into a food adventure

IAN BIRCH

IB
Dec '25

"A Diet You Can Live With – Turning the quest for vitamins, proteins, antioxidants, phytochemicals, prebiotics, fibers and more, into a food adventure", **Book 1 of the series** by Ian Birch.

ISBN: 978-1-0686374-2-1

Cover designed by Getcovers. See: https://getcovers.com/

DISCLAIMERS

Always consult your doctor. If you are in any doubt regarding your health, then consult your doctor before making any changes to your lifestyle including diet or exercise and please follow their advice.

The information presented in this book is for educational purposes only. This should not replace advice from a qualified medical professional and does not offer medical advice as I am not a medical doctor or nutritionist. The information in this book is based on my own personal experiences and on my own interpretation of research and other available sources.

This book is for healthy adults. The information in this book is intended for healthy adults. If you have any concerns regarding your health, you must consult your doctor and follow their advice.

This book does not offer guaranteed outcomes. The book describes outcomes Ian Birch experienced personally. The outcomes for anyone following any of the suggestions and ideas expressed within will vary for many reasons and so the outcomes cannot be guaranteed. Ian Birch does not assume liability for any injuries, personal loss, or illness caused using this information.

Keep this fun and enjoyable. It is the intention of the author to provide ideas and suggestions anyone can use to experiment and explore the food they buy in order to modify and improve their regular diet. The ideas and suggestions are presented in ways that are easy to adapt to just about any individual lifestyle and can be used across a range of personal food preferences. And most importantly, the author found that making his own regular diet fun and enjoyable played an important part in his own successful outcomes and encourages you to do the same.

.

CONTENTS

Acknowledgements

I must start by saying thank you to my family for bearing with me over the years as I headed off in all sorts of directions in my research. And for their encouragement to put pen to paper and the ongoing support to complete what turned out to be a much larger task than first appeared.

Special thanks must also go to Dr Younis, the Harley Street Specialist to whom I owe so much. His patience, curiosity and perseverance helped me through a difficult time. Unfortunately, we lost contact, and I was so sad to hear that he had passed away before he could see the fruits of our joint endeavour. I remain forever grateful.

I must also thank my good friend Alan Watson, otherwise known as "Alan the Artist" for his numerous sketches that livened up the original notes and some of which now live on in the final work.

And a quick note about spelling. I am used to spelling certain words a little differently. For example, I generally write Fiber as Fibre so that is how you might find it in the text. There are other words that might differ too. Sometimes I might use an "s" for "z", "ou" for "o" or abbreviations such as Carbs, Veg and Veggies. So can I ask that you bear with me.

Finally, I would like to thank the various sources I have used to illustrate important points or provide various data or concepts. And I will finish by stating that any errors, mistakes or omissions are mine and mine alone.

1. Introduction

The food we eat should both nourish the body and fuel us up for life. And yet for many of us it can be quite a challenge to follow a healthy diet despite all the advice and options available.

For a start, how do you even begin to choose from the vast array of foods available now? The choices can be overwhelming. And how can you make sense of all the messages and advice about which are the best foods to eat, and which are the healthiest choices? Especially when those messages and advice are often confusing and even conflicting.

And there's more. What about all the different nutrients we need to cover? We might be familiar with our Proteins, Carbohydrates and Fats as well our Vitamins, Minerals and Water, and possibly our Fibres too. But that list is expanding to include Antioxidants and Phytochemicals, Probiotics and Prebiotics. Where do we find these in our diet?

Plus, there are all sorts of reasons any of us might seek to improve our diet. For example, you might be looking to improve your diet to take care of your health, lose a bit of weight, regain your old energy, or rebuild your fitness and even put on a bit of weight as you get stronger.

Or maybe you are looking after the diet of your family, trying to work out how to cater for all sorts of different requirements and preferences.

You may well have read up on all sorts of "special diets" and might now be wondering why or how this is different.

Well, the purpose of this book is to provide a framework that just about anyone can use, regardless of food preferences, to experiment, explore and improve their diet. This framework uses 3 Diet Hacks that show how we can all strive to include all the nutrients we need and in roughly the right portion sizes and ratios to fit with our individual lifestyles.

But the framework doesn't rely on exotic "superfoods" that will magically change your life or on cutting out every food you like and living on a couple of lettuce leaves and 5 gallons of water.

The framework helps you pick out the best foods you can buy locally, which could be at the supermarket, the local shops or even local farm shops if there are any close by. There are plenty of good foods, great foods even, and the framework and 3 Diet Hacks show you how to experiment and explore the different foods to make the most of them.

So yes, this book is for any adult looking to get the absolute most from the food they eat every day. But really, the book is more like a quest or a journey of discovery, exploring the foods you already eat as well as new foods that maybe you haven't considered before. And you can re-visit favourite meals, dishes and recipe books. There are all sorts of ways you can start to improve your diet every day.

Also, rather than worrying about restricting or cutting specific foods out and all that sort of stuff, we are going to turn your food back into an adventure by working out the foods you can choose to eat every day to provide all the nutrients and nourishment you need to live your life to the full.

And this journey starts with understanding how food actually works, or rather how the different nutrients work. And how the body works. Then we work out where to find these nutrients in the foods you can buy locally so that you too can build a diet that powers you up for life.

On my own journey back to good health and fitness I had to try and find out why different nutrients were important and how they worked before I felt confident about adjusting and fine tuning my own diet. I enjoyed the whole process of researching and testing. I still do.

So, if you want to find out how your nutrients can work for you and how you can start getting the absolute most from the food you eat every day, then join me on the journey to build:

A Diet You Can Live With.

Starting out with 3 Guidelines

My own journey started in the late 1980s as I struggled to recover from a severe tropical illness that eventually left me totally incapacitated for over two years. Then I was lucky to team up with Dr Younis, a Harley Street Specialist, and with his help my health finally started to turn around. As I emerged from those years and slowly rebuilt my health and fitness again, I tried to make sense of the advice I was given by several clinical dieticians. This advice included 3 Guidelines as follows:

- Aim for 2,500 calories a day.
- Mix your Macros: Carbs 50% | Fats 35% | Proteins 15%
- Eat 5 portions of fruit & veg a day.

But these guidelines are so generalized that they didn't really provide a framework I could use every day and so I floundered. But once again Dr Younis took up the challenge, and together we unpicked these guidelines and took everything back to the base nutrients. As soon as we did this everything changed.

Making Food an Adventure Again

I was off on a journey of discovery and what a journey. Well, more like an adventure and the best way to sum it up is with the 6 Parts that make up the book as follows:

> **Part 1 – 3 Diet Hacks that can work for just about anyone.** We explore how they came about, why they can work for just about anyone and encourage you to embrace the challenge to keep exploring. Your food should be an adventure.
>
> **Part 2 – The Base Nutrients we all know.** Well, I thought I knew about Vitamins, Minerals, Proteins, Carbs and Fats, but when you start delving deeper there is so much more to them
>
> **Part 3 – The Missing Nutrients we need to know more about.** These are the nutrients, including Soluble & Insoluble Fibres Antioxidants & Phytochemicals, Probiotics & Prebiotics, that our body uses in slightly different ways. They facilitate or enable vital functions and so I call them my Vital Nutrients. And this is the most exciting area of the whole book
>
> **Part 4 – The Foods we eat.** We take a tumbling ride through the evolution of the human diet, from the hunter gatherer diet

of our distant ancestors through to the modern farmer diet. We humans are creative, finding all sorts of ways to produce edible foods from different sources, and different physical environments. Maybe we can take a fresh look at how we can make the absolute most of some of the new foods in our diet.

Part 5 – The Calorie Conundrum and our Macronutrients. Let's pull apart all these slogans like Low Fat, No Fat, Low Carb or High Protein Diets. The simple truth is that not all of your daily calories are used for energy, so let's explore how to get the most from your macronutrients.

Part 6 – How 3 Diet Hacks can provide all our nutrients. Through the book we seem to be building what seems like an ever-expanding list of nutrients we all need to try to include in our diet. And yet the 3 Diet Hacks provide a framework just about anyone can use to cover all their nutrients.

The Small Intestine, the Microbiome and our Vital Nutrients

I must expand on Part 3 where we explore topics as diverse as:

- An overlooked physical aspect of the small intestine and why our fibres have such a huge impact on our digestion.
- How the Microbiome in our Small and Large Intestines plays such an important role in our digestion.
- How the Microbiome or Gut Flora in the small intestine impacts on our overall health, can trigger our moods and even affect our immune system, leading some to describe this combination with the Small Intestine as our "Second Brain".

For me this is the most exciting aspect of our diet. I refer to the nutrients that have such an impact on these areas of our digestion and overall health as Vital Nutrients.

The Vital Nutrients are the "extras" like our Fibres, Antioxidants and Phytochemicals. And some perform more than one role. For example, some Fibres help facilitate physical aspects of our digestion and others act as Prebiotics feeding our Microbiome.

And the research on the Microbiome is so exciting. The emerging science is completely redefining our understanding of the human condition.

3 Guidelines become 3 Diet Hacks

I cannot hide the fact that some Sections will be heavy going. Nor can I hide the fact that the story weaves one way and another.

So, this Book takes you on a helter-skelter ride breaking our diet down to **the base nutrients we all need**. Then it puts it all back together again in 3 Diet Hacks that just about anyone can use regardless of any food preferences. And the 3 Diet Hacks are:

- Eat a variety of fresh non-starchy veg in 4 generous portions and fruit in modest portions.
- Count my proteins (and include wide variety)
- Plan my meals (to cover my optimum energy calories each day)

At first glance they might look a lot like the three Guidelines I started with, but the secret is in the detail and the order.

Once you strip everything back to the base nutrients we all need, which we will call our Food Types, then everything changes. The 3 Diet Hacks provide a framework that I can adapt to suit whatever life is throwing at me or whatever it is I want to achieve. My diet isn't a chore, it is an adventure. And now you can join me on that adventure.

This Book can never be finished!

My journey started way back in the late 1980s:

- Before the re-instatement of the ORAC Test for Antioxidants (2013)
- Before the Human Microbiome Project (2007-2012)
- Before the internet even (back in the last century)

I have found myself drawing on the lessons of the past and interpreting them in the light of emerging science.

I find it encouraging that empirical observations of personal health benefits in those early years seem to be supported by the emerging science in the intervening years.

And yet my 3 Diet Hacks have provided me with a framework that allows this to happen, well actually they encourage it. My diet doesn't stand still, there are new foods to discover, new preparations and combinations to test out.

But this Book is really about You

My diet is the food I eat to keep fit and healthy and to power my life. It is certainly a Diet I can Live With.

But we are all different. Yes, we need the same base nutrients but how our bodies work with different foods will vary from one person to another.

Whilst acknowledging that we all make choices based on budget, availability, preferences or beliefs, we must still seek to find foods that provide the nutrients we need, that we can readily digest and that are enjoyable to eat.

I had a big incentive to experiment and explore my own diet and to be honest, it was quite awkward at first. But in the end, I was genuinely surprised at how my whole view of food changed. Now I look at my food in terms of how it can provide the nourishment I need, then I seek out the nourishing foods I enjoy eating. My food is fun and enjoyable, and I find myself eating in elegant sufficiency.

Now I hope I can encourage you to explore your food options with an open mind and take your own journey to find what works for you and to build:

A Diet You Can Live With

Part 1 – 3 Diet Hacks that can work for just about anyone

2. Why the 3 Diet Hacks can work for anyone

But we are all different!

In the context of diet, nutrition, health and fitness I would hazard a guess that most people would initially think about our differences in terms of:

- Body size & shape
- Level of activity
- Metabolism
- Gender & Age
- Lifestyle
- And possibly Food preferences

And in today's connected world we are probably much more aware of even more differences.

Now going back a few years, before the internet even, I was lucky enough to live and work in half a dozen countries around the world and travel extensively in many others.

I've mingled with people of all sorts of different ethnicity, culture, religion, belief, levels of wealth and lifestyles. Their food choices may be determined by:

- food preferences
- beliefs and conscience
- financial constraints
- culture

- geographic location
- food allergies or intolerances
- personal motivation/limitations/necessity

And yet despite all these differences I still maintain that my 3 diet hacks can work for just about anyone.

Our differences are something to celebrate

As a result of my own travels, I became aware that some people hold strong views about how they and others live their lives. But I have a request please:

Can we acknowledge our differences and give each other a bit of slack?

Because as we live our lives, we all leave a "footprint" on this planet. Yes, each and every one of us. And despite all our differences, I truly believe that most people really are just trying to live their lives as best they can.

Indeed, we can look back into our distant past and see that so many of our own species, the *Homo sapiens,* were doing just that as they adapted to all sorts of environments around the world.

And both our distant ancestors and our current neighbours found and continue to find all sorts of ways to survive and thrive in a huge range of climates, landscapes and even seascapes.

Perhaps the most remarkable achievement is that we humans have found any number of ingenious ways to change previously inedible foods into staple foods for whole populations around the world.

And now it seems that we are becoming more aware of the impact we are having on the planet. This is changing how we view each other and the world around us.

As you are reading this book, I'd like to suggest that we all try to do more for ourselves, for each other, our families, our communities and the planet for which we are all responsible.

So, let's treat this multi-faceted progress, the diversity and all the resulting differences as something to celebrate.

Indeed, it seems that there are so many ways that we are different…

…AND YET we all need the same Base Nutrients

This might seem like a rather bold statement, but this is one simple truth that seems to be lost in all the human diversity and in the dizzy array of diet and nutrition options we are bombarded with.

And it is a hard truth I had to find out the hard way.

But when you cut everything back to the base nutrients, find out how food works and how your body uses these nutrients, then everything changes.

Because the 3 Diet Hacks do just that they provide a framework to build a "Balanced Diet" to suit just about anyone:

- Slimmers
- Athletes
- Omnivores
- Carnivores
- Vegetarians
- Vegans
- Pescatarians
- Families
- Workaholics
- Party Goers
- In fact, just about anyone

Despite all our differences we also have so much in common, we all need the same base nutrients. And so, the next big question is:

Where do we find all the base nutrients that we need in the food choices we have?

The choices we make may be partly determined for us by factors such as our location, culture and finances. Or we may determine them by our conscience, beliefs and lifestyle.

So, as we set off to explore how you can build "a diet you can live with" it is important to remember that:

We are all human.

and

We all need the same base nutrients.

3. How the 3 Diet Hacks came about

An active life

I should tell you a bit about me. Back in my youth I did love my sport. As a kid Swimming & Tennis were my thing. I also got into hiking and through my teens I started hiking in my local hills and gradually moved on to hiking in the mountains.

In amongst all this, when I was 11 years old (which I will write as @11from now on) I got involved in Coastal Rowing but only as a cox because I was "small". But I was hooked on rowing and @18 despite still being "too small" I went for it and won my novices.

What a stroke of luck because just a few weeks later I went off to university at Imperial College of Science and Technology London. I signed up to row as soon as I got there. And because I had won my novices, I had to join the senior squad.

Happy days! Despite still being on the small side for rowing I made the first VIII all three undergraduate years winning at HRR in 1978.

On graduation I was torn. Much as I loved my sport, my whole life plan was to get into mineral exploration and venture out to the remotest, wildest places in the world. I gave up the sport with some reluctance and plunged headlong into the world of exploration.

Off I went, deserts in the Middle East, jungles in PNG, the never-ending Australian outback and even the Arctic Circle. Yet more Happy Days! Even now I still have to pinch myself at just how lucky I was. I got to see some fantastic parts of the world and mix with all sorts of different cultures and people.

And right up to this point I should add that I didn't really take any notice of my diet. I just ate everything in sight. I could eat 5 meals a day but because I was so active, I stayed lean & fit.

But my world came crashing down.

In my late 20s I picked up a tropical illness working in mangrove swamps in Papua New Guinea, but it was mis-diagnosed. I appeared to recover but it came back to bite again a few years later.

When it did come back to bite me, it hit me hard. By the age of 32 I was a physical wreck and had to leave mineral exploration and the life I loved because I couldn't cope with the rigours anymore.

My health continued to deteriorate, and my body wasted away. Indeed, for quite some time my weight hovered around or even dropped below 8 stone. That is less than 112 lbs. or 50 kg. Look, I am a little over 5' 11" or 181 cm so I was quite literally like a bag of bones.

Specialists, Dietary Advice and 3 Guidelines

Over the next two years and more I was shuffled from one specialist to the next, first in Australia and then back in the UK. As the months and then years went by, I became desperate to find a way to recover my health and fitness.

None of the various specialists were able to diagnose the problem. However, three of them did send me off to see their respective qualified clinical dietitians to try and address the massive weight loss. Each time, I was given what can only be described as the "regular" dietary advice.

The term "balanced diet" came up again and again together with all sorts of "guidelines" including three in particular and in this specific order:

1. Aim for 2,500 calories a day.
2. Mix your Macros: Carbs 50% | Fats 35% | Proteins 15%
3. Eat 5 portions of fruit & veg a day.

As I was starting out, the third of these was more like "eat a variety of fruit & veg every day" and this evolved into the familiar "5 a day" guideline now recommended by the World Health Organization and other similar organizations. The other two guidelines are also from reputable sources which I will come back to in due course.

But without a framework to implement these "guidelines" I floundered and made little progress.

It looked like I was condemned to spend the rest of my life living off pills and shakes.

My Lucky Break

By pure luck I ended up with a Harley Street specialist, Dr Younis. He took a completely different approach and set about trying to work out why I couldn't absorb food properly.

In the simplest possible terms, he diagnosed that the tropical illness had completely disrupted my small intestines. His treatment stabilized the small intestines and he then dealt with the other complications, one requiring minor surgery. It was all a bit messy really, so I shan't go into detail.

Dr Younis was turning my health predicament around and my life finally turned a corner too. I was on the mend even though I was still living on pills and shakes. The shakes were the only food I seemed to be able to digest and absorb.

The next stage was working out how I could get back to "normal" foods. It was a real struggle, but I didn't want to spend the rest of my life living off pills and shakes. He was very patient as he worked with me to find a way forward using and developing those 3 guidelines into a framework that I could use every day.

Perhaps the reason we got on so well was that we were both curious. We both wanted to explore how to build a diet that worked for me again.

It wasn't a case of just challenging the orthodoxy for the sake of it. It was about taking generalized advice like the three guidelines and finding ways to make them work. Providing that missing framework if you like.

Sadly, Dr Younis died a few years later but I shall always be grateful for his, patience, guidance and commitment to my recovery. But the seeds of my 3 diet hacks were sown and I was on my way again.

3 Guidelines become 3 Diet Hacks

Now the next turn of events was not quite as dramatic. I got married and started a family. You can just get swept up with it all. Well, I did!

But what a time?

And I must say that we had some fun with the kids helping them explore and enjoy their food. My wife and I used to chuckle when they had friends around and the parents were astonished that somehow their children had joined the fun devouring cucumber, carrots, broccoli and all sorts of foods they would barely touch at home.

Anyway, the years flew by but as I approached the point when the last of the kids (a term of affection, honestly) was heading off to university I realized that I had forgotten to look after myself. **Oh dear!**

Although I had enjoyed reasonable health for years, with no more serious illness to speak of, it started to dawn on me that I was a real mess. I had a horribly bulging waist, had no energy, no strength, just doing day-to-day stuff was a struggle.

It is a funny thing, isn't it? You make sure everyone else is getting their nutrition, their rest and so on but just sort of forget about yourself.

As my 55th birthday came and went in 2013, I took a long hard look at myself and realized I had let my own good eating habits slip away.

I needed to change, so at 55 (@55) I set about applying my diet habits again. I went right back to my days with Dr Younis.

Keeping it all as simple as possible, I refined all my notes into 3 simple diet hacks that I follow to this day:

- Eat a variety of fresh non-starchy veg in 4 generous portions and fruit in modest portions.
- Count my proteins (and include wide variety)
- Plan my meals (to cover my optimum energy calories each day)

At first glance these apparently simple hacks just look like a variation of the three guidelines mentioned earlier. But they are considerably more than that. The secret is in the detail and the re-jigged order.

Everything Changes with the Base Nutrients

On my journey with Dr Younis, I had to break everything back down to the base nutrients. This was a revelation.

Once you understand how your body utilizes the base nutrients then everything changes.

Now that I was using my 3 Diet Hacks again, I started to continuously fine tune them to keep them easy and fun. It didn't take long to start turning things around.

A Good Outcome

I finally got serious again and started using the 3 diet hacks properly. And as 2013 rolled into 2014, I lost over 17lbs in just 14 weeks, mostly that awful subcutaneous fat bulging around the waist. I was getting stronger and fitter again. Then my life took off:

> @56 I qualified as a Firefighter with my local Fire & Rescue Service
>
> @57 I raced my first Tough Mudder and went hiking in the mountains again
>
> @58 I raced a rowing VIII again in the Vets Head
>
> @60 I completed RatRace for the first time
>
> @61 I completed my first Spartan Race. Well, I was running it rather than racing and I did mess up tackling a couple of obstacles.
>
> @62 I was still going strong in the Fire & Rescue Service and planning to actually race my next Spartan Event

As 2020 unfolded and @62 I had to accept that my eyes were now a bit of an issue or could become an issue. Nothing serious but it could impact on my ability to see clearly in a difficult situation like poor light. Just an age thing, I guess. So, I left the Fire and Rescue Service before it became a problem and decided to start a new chapter.

Unfortunately, this coincided with all the COVID business and what a terrible time that was. But even so, after hanging up my Firefighter

Helmet for the last time I was reflecting on how my life had turned around since my 55th birthday.

My hectic schedule of work as a Firefighter, busy family life, plenty of social activity and all the fun stuff, it was all powered by my 3 diet hacks!

The Seed was Sown

As I was looking through the notes, I had kept over the years I got to thinking that I should compile them into a more reader friendly version for anyone else who might be interested.

I was reluctant at first, but a few people kept prompting me. My kids for a start. They had all grown up loving their fruit & veg and had gone on to follow three completely different diet paths in terms of protein preferences.

In addition, a few of the parents of Juniors I had coached at rowing enjoyed the various notes I provided on nutrition and were still curious to find out more. And there were a few friends who just wanted to know how I seemed to keep in shape without any apparent effort.

I was still exploring and researching a range of nutrition related topics as well. And the more I explored the diet hacks, the more I felt they could apply to just about anybody.

Well, I keep saying that the framework and 3 Diet Hacks can work for just about anyone. So, I should start by explaining how I have used the same framework to achieve three quite different objectives:

1. Regaining lost weight after illness
2. Losing excess weight following years of sedentary living and poor diet
3. Maintaining optimal weight, and more specifically an optimal waistline, through the ebb and flow of life

But to explain that I need to explain the difference between Weight Loss and Fat Loss and the importance of the Waistline.

4. Weight Loss, Fat Loss and Your Waistline

Weight loss is a big issue and it may affect more of us than we might care to admit. In 2013 I didn't recognise that I had an issue, so the reality came as a shock. Over the years I had tried to follow a diet to build and maintain an optimal body weight, but as I found out, body shape and the waistline are more important health indicators.

Now, back in Chapter 3 I explained how in the beginning I was using my diet to rebuild my health and **gain** body weight lost through illness.

Then more recently I started following the 3 Diet Hacks properly again. For various reasons I had let my diet slip, and I was combining my refreshed diet with a gentle exercise regime to lose a bit of excess weight. I only expected to lose maybe 5-6 lbs but ended up losing over 17lbs over a 14-week period.

In order to explain the difference between the anticipated outcome and the actual outcome experienced over that 14-week period I need to compare two different health measures.

And I must make clear that I am not offering medical advice here. If you are seeing your doctor for a check-up then you can always discuss the information with them as well. It is your health data after all.

Body Mass Index v Waist to Height Ratio

The Body Mass Index is a health measure or screening tool used as a matter of course by health professionals here in the UK. It is also widely used in many other countries including the USA.

The Body Mass Index is a simple calculation using a person's height and their weight. The person's weight in kilograms is divided by their height in metres squared. A score of 18.5 - 24.9 is considered healthy.

A score of 25 or more is considered overweight. Starting out my Body Mass Index score came in around 23 which was deemed to be healthy, but indicated I was maybe a few lbs, say 5-6 lbs, over my ideal weight.

But the Body Mass Index measure is a bit of a conundrum. It is a useful tool to measure whole populations but is less useful on a personal level. This conundrum is explained quite elegantly by Cathy O'Neil in her book *Weapons of Math Destruction* (p 176). She writes:

> *This (the Body Mass Index) is based on a formula devised two centuries ago by a Belgian mathematician, Lambert Adolphe Jacques Quetelet, who knew next to nothing about health or the human body. He simply wanted an easy formula to gauge obesity in a large population. He based it on what he called the "average man".*

Weapons of Math Destruction (Cathy O'Neil, 2016), see **Ref 1**

It has always struck me as odd that a tool specifically developed "to gauge obesity in a large population" ends up being used as a personal health measure. But this conundrum might explain my own personal observations because whilst my Body Mass Index score only indicated a modest problem, my Waist to Height Ratio indicated a rather more pressing problem. So, what is the Waist to Height Ratio?

The Waist to Height Ratio may be referred to as WtHR and may also be called the Waist to Stature Ratio or WSR. I will stick to Waist to Height Ratio.

This is probably the simplest body measurement you can take, well two measurements, your waist and your height. The Ratio is simply the Waist measurement divided by the Height measurement, and the Ratio might well be the most useful personal health measure to monitor.

Measuring your height is straightforward but we should clarify how to measure the circumference of your waist.

As a general guide I would say that for most of the people I have tried this on it usually means the tape measure is 1-2 inches above the belly button. But because this is so important I refer to The World Cancer Research Fund who suggest the method shown in **Fig 1** over the page and see **Online Source 1.**

The reason this Waist measurement is so important is because the level of Belly Fat or subcutaneous fat we see around the waist is indicative of the level of intra-abdominal or Visceral fat deep within the abdomen. High levels of Visceral Fat can be one of the main indicators of increased risk of a host of diseases including High Blood Pressure, Heart Attack and Diabetes.

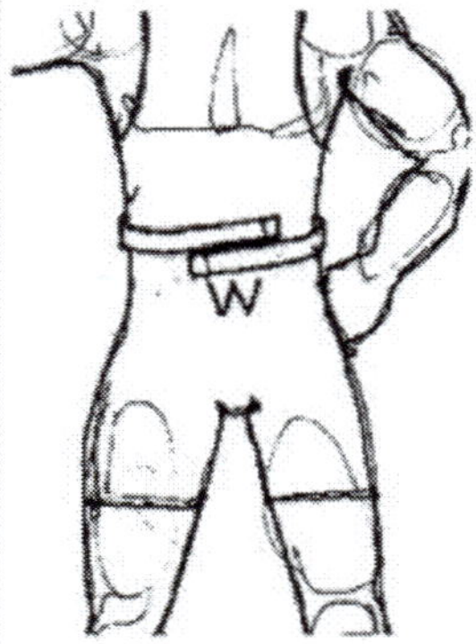

1 Place the tape measure around your waist, at the halfway point between the bottom of your lowest rib and the top of your hip bone. If you have trouble finding this point, then lean to one side and see where the skin folds. This is the point where you can measure your waist.

2 Make sure it's level and a snug fit, but not digging into your skin.

3 Breathe normally, and measure after you have breathed out.

Fig 1. Measuring the Waist

There is an important difference between the BMI Score and the Waist to Height Ratio.

The BMI Score gives a general indication of the level of fat throughout the body but doesn't identify where it is. But the Waist to Height Ratio is specifically identifying the level of the key Visceral Fat deep in the abdomen. And this deep visceral fat is a big health indicator.

Elizabeth Blackburn, Nobel Prize winner, and Elissa Epel, in their wonderful book *The Telomere Effect*, sum it as follows:

> *Subcutaneous fat, found under the skin and in the limbs, carries fewer health risks. High intra-abdominal fat is metabolically troublesome and indicates some level of poor glucose control or insulin resistance.*

The Telomere Effect (Elizabeth Blackburn and Elissa Epel, 2017), see **Ref 2**

By intra-abdominal fat, they mean the deep-seated Visceral Fat.

Other widely used health measures include the Waist Circumference and Waist to Hip Ratio. Whilst they all provide useful information about our state of health, only the Waist to Height Ratio provides a measure with universal application, as described below:

> *The waist-height ratio (WtHR) stood out in recent years as a measure that allows correction for the stature of each individual thus a single threshold could be identified and unified for all ethnic groups in different populations and in both sexes. A systematic review and metaanalysis revealed a value of 0.5 to be of global application to identify an increased cardiovascular and metabolic risk.*

Alaa Youssef Ahmed Ahmed Baioumi, in Nutrition in the Prevention and Treatment of Abdominal Obesity (Second Edition), 2019.

See *Online Source 2

The universal rule is that 0.5 is the key marker. Less than this and your health risks are low, greater than this and the risks start increasing. And this illustrates the importance of our body shape as shown in **Fig 2** below.

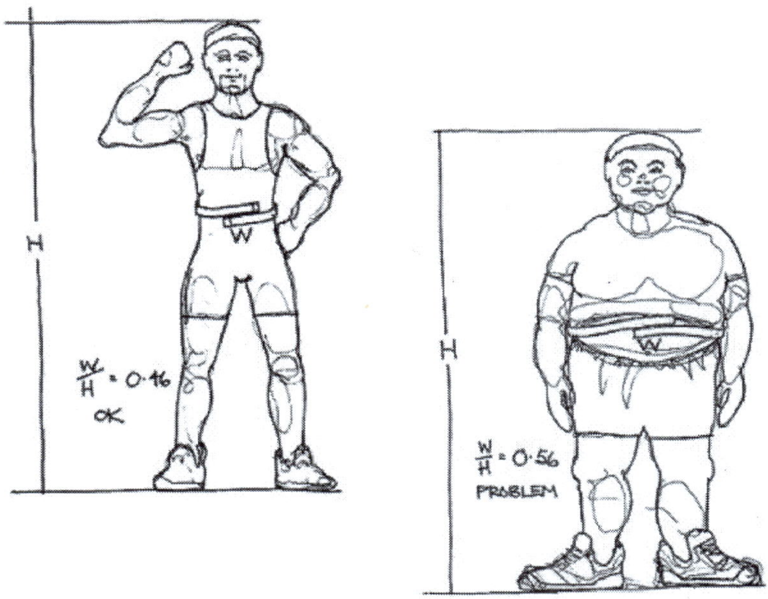

Fig 2. Waist to Height Ratio

This is still inexact though because our natural body shapes, the optimal body shape defined by our DNA, will vary from one person to the next.

I am naturally slim so anything above 0.5 screams a warning. For someone with a naturally bigger or bulkier build has a bit more leeway. But the value of 0.5 as the turning point works for everyone. This is the key marker.

In my case, my overall body weight did appear to only be a few pounds over my supposedly ideal weight. And yet I had lost weight, or rather muscle mass from my arms, legs and shoulders. But I had put on weight as fat around my waistline and deep in the abdomen.

So, my arms, legs and shoulders were thinner than they used to be, and my waistline had **expanded (a lot).**

This in turn revealed a universal truth about our skeletal muscles:

Use them or lose them

We all have to work our muscles to build and maintain our muscle mass and keep them all in good working order. That includes the big muscles we can see in our arms and legs, the stabilizer muscles that keep complicated joints like the shoulders and knees in good working order and the deeper muscles like the core muscles that hold the spine in place and keep it strong and flexible.

If you don't look after your muscles, they lose both their strength and their mass. In other words, they shrink. The BMI score masked this situation, but the Waist to Height Ratio revealed it.

Now the long-term outcome was that after losing over 17 lbs, I then put most of that weight back on again. But this time I was rebuilding that lost muscle mass in my arms, legs, shoulders and core. Over the subsequent years my weight has varied depending on the type of exercise I was doing. Sometimes I have even weighed a bit more than when I started.

I'm not talking about turning into a bodybuilder, I'm not even talking about some ideal weight, rather I am talking about finding my optimal body shape and in particular, an optimal waistline.

So, my waist dropped from over 37" to ~ 33". And this meant that my Waist to Height Ratio dropped from over 0.52 to ~0.47, comfortably below that 0.5 marker. With very little effort, it has remained around that mark ever since.

Now I am not particularly fussed about having "ripped abs", but I do like having a well-defined waist.

So, whilst it is important to monitor weight and weight loss, I suggest that changing body shape, specifically losing abdominal fat and aiming for a well-defined waist is a more useful and more satisfying measure to pursue.

Fat Loss, Body Shape and Waistlines

At the beginning of this Chapter I suggested that Weight Loss, or rather the need to Lose Weight, affects more of us than we might like to admit. Now I can explain what I mean. Or rather I can ask:

> **"How many people who believe they are close to their optimal weight or maybe a few pounds over, might then use the Waist to Height Ratio and find that they have lost muscle mass through inactivity and masked this with excess fat, especially around the waist?"**

It is not a lot of, or even just a bit of "Extra Weight" that is the problem. Having "Too Much Fat" is the real problem and this is especially so when considering the deep visceral fat in the abdomen which is a clear marker of increasing health risk. Now excess fat on the hips or the back of the arms might be rather unsightly, but it is the deep visceral fat and bulging waistline that is the real health marker.

So, the real goal here is "Fat Loss" and especially **"Fat Loss from the Waistline".** And the Waist to Height Ration gives us all a great tool to monitor the waistline, the deep visceral fat and hence our health.

Now it might be puzzling how the diet I describe in this book has served three quite different objectives:

1. Regaining lost weight after illness
2. Losing excess weight following years of sedentary living and poor diet
3. Maintaining optimal weight, and more specifically an optimal waistline, through the ebb and flow of life

But that gets right to the heart of the matter. You see the framework and the 3 Diet Hacks help me to eat a wide selection of foods, especially ones I enjoy, but always in elegant sufficiency.

And I know that most days I will cover all the nutrients I need. But on the days when I don't manage that, well it's just not a problem because I can get back on track as quickly as I like.

There is another surprising benefit. If your diet provides all the different nutrients you need, in foods the body is designed to digest and process, then it does start looking after itself. In fact, you may even find yourself actively seeking out those foods in preference to the junk foods that line so many shelves of every supermarket. It just happens.

Naturally I check my weight from time to time. But the easiest measure of how well I am doing is the waistline. If I have strayed a bit from my ideal diet, then that is where it shows. So, I just give myself a bit of a reminder and put a bit more emphasis on my non-starchy veggies and my proteins. They are the foods that really nourish and satiate. And as it happens, they are the foods I enjoy the most. So, it's a win-win situation.

And now before we can move on, I need to explain or rather untangle some of the terminology around our food and our nutrition.

5. Untangling terminology to get the most from this book

As soon as you step into the "world of diet" you are bombarded with terminology. Some of the terminology is scientific, some is not. It can be very confusing and intimidating. But don't be put off by this. In fact, I strongly recommend embracing it.

Indeed, getting to grips with the scientific terminology will help you develop your knowledge of the building blocks of good nutrition and the confidence to build your own diet.

This book introduces you to key terminology and aims to provide some context to help make some of the more complicated issues a little easier to understand and apply.

All sorts of questions

I must admit when I started on my own journey it was daunting. Just as I was getting a grip on one issue, another came into view, then another. It was frustrating at first. But I embraced the process of exploring the subject and over time my own list of questions steadily grew, covering issues like:

How many calories do I really need? – pp 38 & 134

Why does the ratio of macronutrients matter? – pp 136 & 144

Where do I find phytochemicals? – pp 81, 93 & 97

Why do I need fibres? – pp 62 & 68

What is my microbiome? – p 73

How do I include all my Vitamins & Minerals? – pp 202 & 245

Why are Vitamins B12 and D so important? – pp 53 & 208

Why are antioxidants important? – pp 81 & 95

Why is the small intestine sometimes referred to as our second brain? – p 76

What does my gut flora do for me? – p 75

Do we all need EPA & DHA for our brains? – pp 48 & 168

Are all saturated fats bad for us? – pp 164 & 212

What are complete proteins? – pp 44, 145 & 225

Why are MCTs (medium chain triglycerides) considered healthy fats? – p 164

Does fruit really make you fat? – p 191

Look, you don't have to know how everything works before you can start applying it. The important thing is to start and then enjoy the journey.

As you progress you will build your knowledge base and your understanding of how the different issues relate and impact on one another. You can focus on the issues or questions that are important to you.

We all need the same base nutrients, our food types, so that is where we begin our journey as students of nutrition. Then our journey will look something like this:

1. Exploring the base nutrients, our **Food Types**

2. Reviewing some aspects of **Human Physiology**

3. Exploring the different foods we eat, the **Food Groups**

4. Developing the **3 Diet Hacks**

The journey weaves it's way between the Types, Physiology and Groups. Then we start bringing them all together using the 3 Diet Hacks. At the end of it all I will cover how just about anyone can use the 3 Diet Hacks to start building your own uniquely balanced diet, a diet that can provide all the nutrients and nourishment you need to live your life to the fullest.

Making the Topics Accessible

As well as presenting the book in 6 Parts described in Chapter 1, the content is also presented with a lot of smallish chapters in order to make all the information and ideas as accessible as possible:

Now I appreciate that everyone has their own approach and that we are all at a different point on our own life journey. You might want to cover the full sweep of topics or have specific topics you want to explore straight away, especially if you find that you are already familiar with some of the early topics, particularly relating to the Food Types.

But even if you are familiar with some topics, I still suggest dipping in just in case there is something new, or a different perspective.

References

I am also sure many of you will want to verify the information and ideas presented here. Or explore some of the topics in more detail. So where appropriate there are references to readily available texts and books on relevant topics.

I have enjoyed following up on some research papers, but I realize that these present a couple of problems:

- It can be difficult to access scientific papers if you are not directly linked to a university or similar research institute.
- The depth of the research can go way beyond what most of us can either understand or readily use.

But there are many readily available online resources published directly by universities, research institutes or other related organizations. There are also reputable online magazines publishing articles by experts in their field.

So, I have included links to a host of reputable resources, sometimes with conflicting views because that is the nature of things. I will do my best to keep the links current but apologies in advance if links change over time.

But most of all I hope this book will give you confidence to use the ideas here to start exploring your own food options and to enjoy your food and as you strive towards a healthy diet to suit your lifestyle.

I love my food and hope together we can turn your food into an adventure and your regular diet into:

A Diet You Can Live With

Seeking Medical Advice

But before we start our study of the Food Types there is one important caveat to consider.

If you are in any doubt about your health, taking any sort of medication or if any ladies are pregnant then you must seek medical advice before making any changes to your diet or embarking on any new exercise activities.

And if you do seek medical advice, then look at this as a positive. You are taking proactive steps to look after your own health and wellbeing.

Getting Started

No matter where you are on your own life journey or how you might choose to study, we can all get started with the building blocks of our regular diet. After all

We are all human
and
We all need the same base nutrients.

So, let's get started with our Base Nutrients.

Part 2 – The Base Nutrients we all know

6. The Base Nutrients - Food Types

Food Types – these are our Base Nutrients

These are the different categories of foods based on their **composition at a molecular level** and **the functions they perform**. The common classification used here in the UK includes **7 Food Types** as follows:

- Proteins
- Carbohydrates
- Fats
- Water
- Minerals
- Vitamins
- Fibres

As we discuss the types in more detail, I will refer to these as **"The 7 Regular Food Types**". But we need to include **two more Food Types**:

- Prebiotics & Probiotics
- Additional Micronutrients including Antioxidants, Phytochemicals and Enzymes

With the exception of water, all the Food Types are then divided into different Sub Types, as explained in due course.

Micronutrients and Macronutrients

Some Food Types such as vitamins and minerals only need to be eaten in small quantities daily or occasionally through any week. These are referred to as our **Micronutrients**.

Proteins, Carbohydrates and Fats on the other hand are Types we need to eat in significant quantities each day. These are referred to as our **Three Macronutrients**.

So Far, So Good

So, we have 9 Food types divided into Micronutrients and Macronutrients. That all seems manageable enough! Let's look a little deeper.

7. Essential and Non-Essential Nutrients

Now we explore the difference between our Essential and Non-Essential Nutrients. This classification can cause some confusion.

All Food Types	Essential Nutrients
Proteins	Proteins (9 or 10 depending on source)
Carbohydrates	
Fats	Fats (2 or 4 depending on source)
Water	Water
Minerals	Minerals (all)
Vitamins	Vitamins (except possibly Vits D & K)
Fibres	
Prebiotics & Probiotics	
Additional Micronutrients including Antioxidants, Phytochemicals & Enzymes	

Table 1. Food Types and Essential Nutrients

The body needs a range of different nutrients to perform all the different functions, and we can obtain all these nutrients through our diet. But the body has the capacity to synthesize some of the nutrients, so it seems we have two different forms of nutrient as follows:

Essential Nutrients

There are chemicals and minerals the body cannot synthesize. These must be ingested through the diet, and hence they are referred to as "Essential Nutrients". So, from the table of Food Types these include:

- Proteins (9 or 10 depending on source)
- Fats (2 or 4 depending on source)
- Water
- Minerals (all)
- Vitamins (all except Vit D and Vit K perhaps?)

We can only obtain these nutrients from the foods we eat and drink. So, we need to include all the essential nutrients in our diet on a regular basis.

Non-Essential Nutrients

The term non-essential may be mis-interpreted to mean that we don't really need these nutrients.

But the term actually means that the body can "convert" other nutrients into the required form. Put another way, the body performs numerous complex functions and can "synthesize" some of the special enzymes and chemicals it requires. These enzymes and chemicals are the non-essential nutrients.

Two Important caveats:

Whilst the body has the capacity to synthesize the non-essential nutrients, it doesn't necessarily have the capacity to produce the full daily requirement.

If we miss any non-essential nutrients from our diet, we need to include more of the essential nutrient or nutrients needed to synthesize them.

So, for example, if there are some non-essential proteins, does this mean we don't really need them in our daily nutrition? Not quite!

Do we need Non-Essential Nutrients in our diet?

As you look down the list of Essential Nutrients on the previous page, it might strike you as odd that one of our key energy sources is missing:

- Carbohydrates

These are not regarded as an "Essential Nutrient" because the body can synthesize the glucose it needs from a range of carbohydrates found in many food groups, from various fats and even proteins.

This serves to illustrate the important point that our bodies do need both the "Essential" and "non-Essential" nutrients. The terminology merely refers to how the body can acquire the different nutrients.

Essential and Non-Essential Proteins

The Proteins are a complex subject which we cover in more detail shortly. It can be quite confusing because it is not the actual proteins that we need to consider in our diet, but the constituent building blocks of all proteins, the amino acids.

Of all the amino acids we require, some are essential and must be included in our diet. Others are non-essential because they can be synthesized in the body.

The confusion can be compounded because different sources identify different numbers of essential and non-essential amino acids. Hence why I have identified there are either 9 or 10 Essential Amino Acids depending on source! The amino Acids are listed in Table 2 on Page 44.

This is just one example where there appears to be conflicting advice. We cover this shortly but just need to appreciate that both nutrition and human physiology are vast subjects, and the science is catching up.

Essential and Non-Essential Fats – a conundrum

As with the Carbohydrates, the fats used or needed for energy are not classified as Essential because they can be sourced from a range of the dietary fats. They can also be synthesized from carbohydrates.

However, the fats in our diet provide more than just energy. For example, some of the different Vitamins we all need are fat soluble. So, we need some fats to provide and store those vitamins.

And yet most sources list just two essential fats, the two polyunsaturated fatty acids:

- Omega 3 Fatty Acid alpha-linolenic acid (ALA)
- Omega 6 Fatty Acid linoleic acid (LA)

But some sources extend this list to four essential fats by including the two specific Long Chain Fatty Acid Omega 3s:

- Eicosapentaenoic Acid (EPA)
- Docosahexaenoic Acid (DHA)

So, should that be 2 Essential Nutrients, or 4? The Essential Fats provide an interesting conundrum further illustrating the point that the science is catching up.

It seems that the Fats, like the Proteins, are a complex subject in their own right so I will come back to them in a later section.

Water is an Essential Nutrient

To highlight the importance of water we just need to remind ourselves that the body of the average adult will be made up of 57-60% water.

It might come as a surprise to find out that the body can actually produce water. It is formed together with carbon dioxide as a by-product of a metabolic process in which oxygen and glucose are used to produce energy.

But the body requires water in large amounts well beyond the body's capacity to produce it and it is therefore defined as an essential nutrient.

Hydration is covered in so many sources I will not expand on it further but will refer to it when relevant.

Essential Vitamins – another conundrum

Our Vitamins are widely researched and reported. They are organic molecules the body needs to perform key functions. Because the body can only utilize small amounts at any time they are classed as micronutrients.

So far so good, but just when we think we understand a Food Type we find:

- Most sources list 13 Vitamins, yet Table 3 on Page 52 shows 15
- Some vitamins are Water soluble, and some are Fat soluble, so we do all need fats in our diet.

The Vitamins also present us with a conundrum because:

- The body can synthesize Vitamins D & K, so are these really "Essential Nutrients"?

We cover more aspects of our Vitamins in Chapter 11. Both the water- and fat-soluble Vitamins are listed and the range of Vitamins we all need highlights the need for diversity of foods in our regular diet.

All Minerals are Essential Nutrients

This might seem obvious, but the body cannot synthesize the individual elements such as Calcium (Ca) Magnesium (Mg) or Zinc (Zn). We all need to include these in our regular diet.

The minerals are also classed as Micronutrients because the body can only utilize small amounts at any time.

We cover more aspects of our Minerals in Chapter 12, including the range of Minerals we all need. Once again, this highlights the need for diversity of foods in our regular diet.

We come back to this issue of diversity again and again on our journey.

So, how does the Body use these Base Nutrients?

We have only covered some of our nutrients so far, but this is an opportune point to consider how the body uses some of these nutrients.

It is important to explore this aspect of nutrition because it highlights that we may need to re-consider how we think some of our nutrients do actually work. There may be some surprises here!

And the best place to start is with the three macronutrients, proteins, fats and carbohydrates and our calorie count.

8. Calories, the Macronutrients and Energy Batteries

Calories and do we really need all that energy?

Our overall nutrition requirements can be defined in terms of the total energy we need each day. This is referred to as the calorie count. The UK government guidelines for the daily calorie count are as follows:

- 2500 calories for the average adult male
- 2000 calories for the average adult female

The equivalent US Government guidelines recommend 2700 and 2200 calories respectively.

However, the Food and Agricultural Organization of the United Nations, (the FAO), calculated the average calorie consumption for the whole populations of the UK and USA. Their figures were 3,440 and 3,700 calories respectively. Does the data suggest a lot of people are eating too much energy?

Macronutrients and our energy requirements

This daily calorie count may also be defined in terms of the ratio of the three macronutrients we need in our diet. In the UK the widely accepted recommendation is:

Carbs 50% | Fats 35% | Proteins 15%*

In other words, 50% of our daily calorie count should be from carbohydrates, 35% from fats and 15% from protein as shown in the online article published by The Faculty of Public Health, **(Online Source 3).** Now the implication of the calorie count as three percentages is that all three of our macronutrients are primarily providing energy. **But is this really the case?**

To make sense of this we need to understand how our macronutrients are used and how our "Energy Batteries" work. We start by considering the main functions of our three macronutrients as follows:

> **Carbohydrates** are the first of our **two main energy sources.** They are broken down to glucose. This provides much of our energy for day-to-day activities. Excess Glucose can be stored, and some is stored as Glycogen. The storage capacity for both is modest and requires **regular topping up through the diet**. Our brain activity uses approximately 20% of our daily glucose.
>
> **Fats** are the second of our **two main energy sources.** We generally think of Fats providing the energy used in **more vigorous short burst activities** or towards the end of longer duration activities. But it is a bit more nuanced than that. Either way, the body stores excess fats for future use in the adipose cells and some organs. The amount of fat we store can be measured in terms of the Body Mass Index, BMI. The body has the **capacity to store a lot of fat.**
>
> **Proteins** can be a source of energy but are **NOT** a primary energy source for the body. The proteins are primarily used for **building and maintaining our skeletal muscle.** In some respects, they are the energy source of last resort when all the other energy sources have been exhausted.

This is not new!

For example, *"The Commando Pocket Manual, 1940-1945"* **(Ref 3)** presents the same calorific ratio for the three Macronutrients. The manual also refers to Fats and Carbs as "fuel foods" and Proteins as "building materials". We will come back to this again in Chapter 27 when we explore "The Calorie Conundrum".

The proteins and some fats also perform a range of other important physiological functions, and we cover these a little later too. But first we need to understand how the body stores and utilizes energy for short term and long-term use.

Your Glucose Battery – short term energy supply

Your body stores a supply of glucose in the bloodstream and stores a variation, glycogen, in the skeletal muscle, the liver, the brain and the kidneys, as shown in Fig 3 below.

We'll call this our "**Glucose Battery**" and this is the first energy source your body will use as you go about your daily life, running all the organs including the brain and your daily activity right up to quite intense endurance activities.

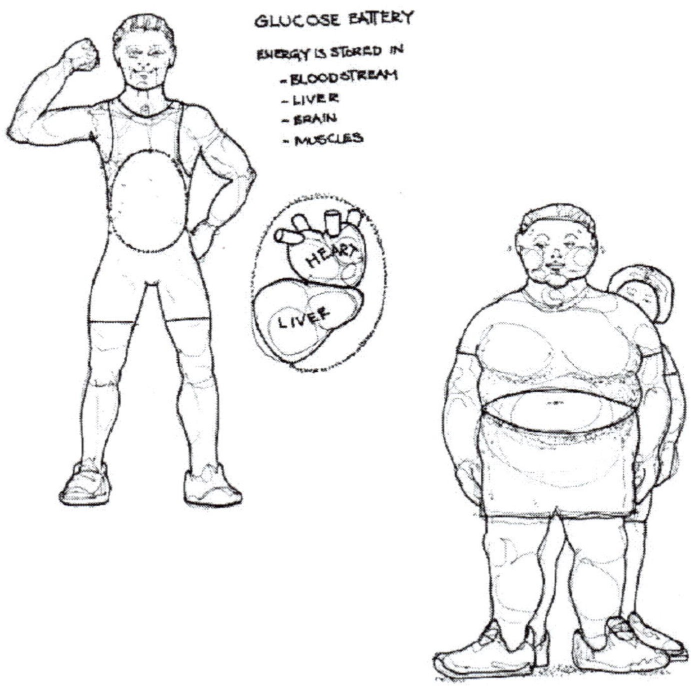

Fig 3. Your Glucose and Fat Batteries

The total storage capacity for your "Glucose Battery" is modest. It is designed to be topped up on a regular basis and when full, excess glucose can be converted to fats.

Your Fat Battery – long term energy supply

The average human has some 30 billion fat cells with three types, white, brown and beige. The total we each have is laid down in adolescence and that number is thought to remain constant throughout our lives. We can accept for the moment that the number of cells remains constant but that the amount of fat each cell stores can vary significantly.

The sub cutaneous fat cells sit just below the skin around areas like the waist, buttocks, thighs and chin shown in **Fig 3** on the previous page. The visceral fat cells sit internally deep within the abdomen and between the various organs. (And I'm sorry, but I didn't want to point to the various places the fat accumulates. You may be like me and might not want to be reminded.)

Excess carbohydrates and even excess proteins from your regular diet can be converted to fats. These together with excess dietary fats can be stored for long term use as Triglycerides in fat cells. A small amount of fat can also be stored in different organs. We'll refer to all this storage as our "**Fat Battery**".

Two Big Problems with your Energy Batteries

It appears that nature has provided an energy storage system that enables us to balance our short term and long-term requirements. However, there is a catch. The Modern Diet combined with **a more sedentary lifestyle** may negate that simple balance.

The first problem seems to be that the Modern Diet provides a lot more energy than many of us need.

It is a pretty safe bet that if you eat more fuel, in other words Carbohydrates and Fats, than your body can use straight away or store for the short term, then some of that excess fuel will be stored in your longer term "Fat Battery". **And your body will just keep storing excess fuel as fat.**

The second problem is that a more sedentary lifestyle can cause us to lose the ability use the stored energy efficiently.

We all have the physical potential to use energy from both our energy batteries. But to keep our energy batteries working at maximum efficiency we need to engage in different levels of physical activity.

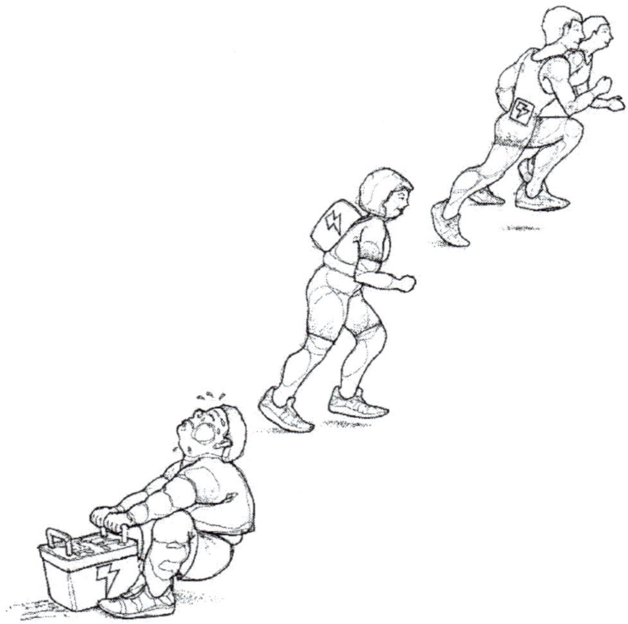

Fig 4. Can you access the energy in your Fat Battery?

So, what happens if you are carrying a lot of stored energy in your Fat Battery and have lost the capacity to use that energy efficiently? It's rather like hauling around a giant spare battery just in case, as in **Fig 4** above. But when you need to use it, it has no charge. Pretty useless really.

A detailed account of the different levels of physical activity is beyond the scope of this book. But we will cover how we can all start to control and then reduce the amount of fat we store in our "Fat Battery" through our diet.

But now we can move onto our Proteins, or more specifically the Amino Acids, and their many functions.

9. Amino Acids and our Proteins

We have talked about the primary role of proteins in terms of building and repairing our skeletal muscles. But there is so much more to them.

The proteins are complex organic molecules and there are literally trillions of them in the human body. The trillions are made up of thousands of different proteins. This is true for both the human body and indeed all living organisms.

Protein molecules are components of every cell in the body, and the thousands of different protein molecules perform or enable all sorts of functions. The proteins can be grouped into categories based on their functions.

Different Protein sub-Types

Some sources list 7 categories, others 9, even 10. I'll use the classification from the University of Utah **(Online Source 4).** We will refer to these 9 categories as our Protein sub-types and they are as follows:

- Enzymes
- Structural Proteins
- Signalling Proteins
- Regulatory Proteins
- Transport Proteins
- Sensory Proteins
- Motor Proteins
- Defence Proteins
- Storage Proteins

It is beyond the scope of this book to describe all the protein sub-Types and their respective functions. But even this simple list highlights the scale and complexity of the proteins in our bodies and their importance in our diet.

Luckily for us we can deal with this scale and complexity by considering the building blocks of all proteins, and these are the Amino Acids.

Amino Acids – the building blocks of all proteins

The thousands of different proteins in our bodies and all living organisms are made up of combinations of amino acids. We humans are made up of Eukaryotic Cells and these are made up of combinations of one or more of **just 20 amino acids of the standard genetic code.**

You might see sources listing 21 or even 22 amino acids. That is because there are two additional rare amino acids, Selenocysteine and Pyrrolysine. However, we will focus on the **20 amino acids** of the standard genetic code. Of these 9 are Essential so we must include them in our diet, and they are listed in Table 2 below.

Essential Amino Acids	Non-Essential Amino Acids
• Histidine	• Alanine
• Isoleucine	• Arginine*
• Leucine	• Asparagine
• Lysine	• Aspartic Acid
• Methionine	• Cysteine
• Phenylalanine	• Glutamic Acid
• Threonine	• Glutamine
• Tryptophan	• Glycine
• Valine	• Proline
	• Serine
	• Tyrosine

Table 2 – Essential and Non-Essential Amino Acids

**From Table 2 - Arginine is an Essential Amino Acid for children but the adult body can synthesize this Amino Acid*

We cover food sources for the amino acids when we cover the concept of "Complete Proteins in Chapter 27.

All the amino acids are literally like building blocks that can be moved around the body to wherever they are needed the most. This attribute is elegantly described by Brad Pilon in his book *"How much protein"*, **(Ref 4).**

We have touched on the classification of nine sub-Types of Proteins. But the story gets more complicated because the amino acids perform additional functions including:

- Proteins, or rather the constituent amino acids are broken down to provide the primary source of Nitrogen (N) for the body.

- There are other organic compounds/molecules in the body that require amino acids. One example, Creatine, is a combination of two Essential Amino Acids and one Non-Essential amino acid.

Scanning Table 2 raises two issues:

- How much protein do we really need?

- How do we include the full range of amino acids in our regular diet?

We start by addressing how much protein we need as a total.

Meeting our Total Daily Protein Requirement

One surprising aspect of the proteins is just how efficiently the body utilizes the amino acids. As a result, our daily requirements are surprisingly modest.

There are several factors to take into consideration in order to estimate our total daily protein requirement and we start to explore these when we look at the Food Groups in Chapter 23. Then in Chapter 27 we look at how we can all count our proteins. This enables us to explore how we can each source our proteins in line with our different food preferences. But the first step is to understand why we all need to take care to cover our total daily protein requirement.

As we explore how to estimate our genuine total daily requirement, we find that exceeding that estimated total protein intake doesn't provide any significant health benefit. However, whilst there is some evidence that eating too much protein may have a detrimental effect on your health, it seems that you would have to eat an awful lot more than you really need for that to be a concern.

Conversely, what happens if we eat too little protein? Perhaps this is an issue that deserves our attention.

But we don't need to get bogged down in that discussion because here and now we can focus on how we can all make a reasonable estimate of an optimal amount of protein to include in our regular diet.

Getting all our Amino Acids is very important

Coming back to the issue of too little protein in our diet, I feel that it is very easy to overlook the importance of the proteins in our diet. As well as aiming for an optimal total daily protein requirement, we also need the full range of all the constituent amino acids.

We all need the full range of amino acids **to build the thousands of different Proteins that** perform all the functions of the different Protein sub-Types, as well as building and maintaining our skeletal muscle mass.

So, I quite deliberately focus on the full range of amino acids and how we can all take reasonable steps to include them all in our regular diet.

Getting all our amino acids is so important and yet I suspect it is an issue that may be glossed over for all sorts of reasons. Throughout this Book I aim to demonstrate that regardless of food preference, omnivore, carnivore, pescatarian, vegetarian or vegan, with a bit of care **we can all do this**.

So, whatever your age or gender, your physical requirements and activity level or your own food preferences, you can enjoy the journey.

10. Essential Fatty Acids and our Brains

There is a lot of confusion around Fats in our diet. Some fats are branded as bad, even dangerous, and there are even calls for "Low Fat" or even "No Fat" diets. Yet other Fats are recognized as healthy, so how can we balance these two issues,

Let's start by considering the many important functions different Fats do perform, in addition to providing energy.

- Fats make up a significant percentage of the brain by weight.
- Fats form part of the membrane in every cell of the body.
- Some of our essential vitamins are Fat soluble.
- Specific fats help clear plaque from the arteries.

The conundrum of 2 or 4 Essential Fats

Despite all the functions of different Fats, many sources list just two Essential Fats, and these are the two polyunsaturated fatty acids:

- Omega 3 Fatty Acid alpha-linolenic acid (ALA)
- Omega 6 Fatty Acid linoleic acid (LA)

But others extend the list to 4 by including two specific Long Chain Fatty Acid Omega 3s:

- Eicosapentaenoic Acid (EPA)
- Docosahexaenoic Acid (DHA)

It is true that the two Long Chain Fatty Acid Omega 3s EPA and DHA can be synthesized from the parent Omega 3 Fatty Acid alpha-linolenic acid or ALA. However, the capacity of the body to synthesize both EPA and DHA seems to vary because of different parameters including gender and age as outlined in the online article published by the Micronutrient Information Center of the Linus Pauling Institute of Oregon State University, **(Online Source 5).**

As a result, many of us for whatever reason will probably not be able to synthesize our full daily requirements of EPA or DHA from ALA. **So, why is this important?**

EPA, DHA, Omega 6 and our Brains

The average adult human brain weighs approximately 3 lbs or 1.36 kg. Approximately 75% of that weight is water. Of the remaining weight some 60% is made up of fats. Some 25% of that fat includes a combination of DHA and the specific derivative of the Omega 6 Arachidonic Acid, AA. Then EPA accounts for up to another 1%.

The high levels of DHA and AA are part of the reason why our brains have been able to develop as they have. The ratio of DHA to AA ranges from approximately 1:1 to 1:2 and together they contribute to the complexity of the possible neural connections and enhanced capacity of the human brain.

The key role the Long Chain Fatty Acid Omega 3 DHA plays in the development of our brains explains why it is so important in our diet.

EPA, DHA, Omega 6 and our Vascular System

Whilst DHA is so important for the brain, the Long Chain Fatty Acid Omega 3 EPA has an equally important role in the vascular system. A combination of EPA and the same Omega 6 derivative AA is found throughout the vascular system together with minor amounts of DHA.

Human Physiology and EPA & DHA

Emerging research also indicates that these two Long Chain Fatty Acid Omega 3s play numerous other key roles in our health. For example, in a paper published on the website of The National Center for Biotechnology Information includes the following:

> *EPA and DHA may affect many aspects of cardiovascular function including inflammation, peripheral artery disease, major coronary events, and anticoagulation. EPA and DHA have been linked to promising results in prevention, weight management, and cognitive function in those with very mild Alzheimer's disease.*

From the paper titled "Omega 3 Fatty Acids EPA and DHA: Health Benefits Throughout Life." By Danielle Swanson. Robert Block and Shaker A. Mousa, **(Online Source 6)**.

It does seem that these two nutrients, DHA and EPA, are very important for our overall health as well as our brain functions.

Seafoods and the Importance of EPA & DHA in our regular diet

There is a growing awareness of the importance of seafoods both in the evolution of humans and in the modern diet. They are the key source of both DHA and EPA across the globe.

In fact, both EPA and DHA are considered so important that respected sources such as the Harvard T.H. Chan School of Public Health in the USA and the NHS in the UK advise people to include portions of fatty fish such as Salmon twice a week.

Indeed, the Harvard T.H. Chan School of Public Health even advises the use of supplements if there is not enough fatty fish in the diet. There are various options with supplements based on Fish, Krill or the longstanding Cod Liver Oil.

Seafoods present a dilemma for vegetarians and vegans. But there is a supplement option based on the algae that the fish and krill feed on.

Other Sources of both EPA & DHA and Omega 6 AA

We live in strange times. Some people still choose to include meat and particularly red meat, in their diet and these foods can be an important source of EPA & DHA. Not as rich a source as seafoods, but still a valuable source, especially from "organ meats" such as liver or kidneys.

Or rather they were, because not so long ago traditionally grazed cattle and sheep provided both EPA and DHA for many people. But modern intense farming methods like increasing the amount of grain in their feed reduced these levels. Indeed, in a lot of cases they are eliminated altogether, a point made eloquently by Lawrence Alderson on page 86 of his book *"The Chance to Survive"*, **(Ref 5).** There is a small but growing body of farmers pursuing "Sustainable or Regenerative" methods and they may also be reviving this source of EPA and DHA.

It is also worth noting that eggs from "free range chickens" can provide EPA and DHA for those vegetarians who choose to eat them, but let's not get drawn into any discussion of food preferences just yet.

It is important to note that many meats, including red meats and other animal products also provide the Omega 6 derivative AA that seems to compliment the DHA and EPA. We will come back to this again.

Even with the very modest trends back to traditional grazing methods and "free range chickens" there is still a persistent message to eat less of these foods, or more specifically to eat less red meat. Are we accidentally excluding key nutrients from our diets?

Omega 3, Omega 6 and our overall Health

We must not forget that the two parent Fatty Acids Omega 3 and Omega 6 perform other important functions. So, we must find ways to include both these Essential Nutrients in our regular diet as well.

What about Non-Essential Fats?

We will come back to other aspects of the Fats in Chapter 28, namely:

- fat soluble vitamins
- short, med & long chain triglycerides
- Too much Omega 6?
- Omega 9
- Saturated Fats and Hydrogenated Oils

But now we can move onto the vitamins.

11. The Essential Vitamins

The correlations between a diet including specific foods like fresh fruits and vegetables, or fish oils like cod liver oil and good health have been recognized across different cultures for many years. But the scientific explanations only emerged with scientific advancements in the 20th century.

As scientific research into poor diet gathered pace, the Swiss chemist Paul Karrer is credited with describing the chemical structure of the first Vitamin which was designated Vitamin A. Two Dutch chemists, David Adriaan van Dorp and Joseph Ferdinand Arens were the first to synthesize Vitamin A in 1947.

Research unlocking the mystery of the different vitamins seemed to tumble out over the following decades. The new discoveries explained anecdotal accounts such as Admiral Nelson insisting on Royal Navy ships carrying fresh fruit and vegetables to counter the risk of scurvy. We now know scurvy is a result of deficiencies in Vitamin C.

Some Northern Europeans used Cod Liver Oil for centuries for protection from the cold and as a remedy for conditions such as rickets. We now know that Rickets is caused by deficiencies in Vitamin D, as reported by Prof George T. Griffing in the Medscape Journal published online in 2008 **(Online Source 7).**

We now also know these oils are a rich source of both Vitamins A and D. So, the cod liver oil helped boost this essential Vitamin D relieving the rickets and Vitamin A helps boost the immune system.

I am sure there are many similar anecdotal accounts from other societies and cultures.

The scientific research in 20th century led to rapid advancements and the creation of a whole new industry providing supplements to boost the health of the wider populations.

There are now many excellent sources of information on our Vitamins and one excellent online source is the Diet and Health Implications for Reducing Chronic Disease Risk published online by the National Library of Medicine **(Online Source 8),** where you can find sections on both Water soluble and Fat Soluble Vitamins I really like the detail in Jane Higdon's book "An Evidence-based Approach to Vitamins and Minerals, Health Benefits and Intake Recommendations, **(Ref 6).**

So rather than trying to replicate those I want to just highlight a few quirks, and a conundrum as follows:

- Many sources list 13 Vitamins, yet others list 15.
- Some vitamins are Water soluble, and some are Fat soluble, so we do need fats in our diet.
- The body can synthesize Vitamins D and K, so are these really "Essential Nutrients"?

The list in Table 3 below has 15 Vitamins. This is because I include the 3 variations of Vitamin B6, pyridoxine, pyridoxal and pyridoxamine.

Water Soluble Vitamins	Fat Soluble Vitamins
• Vit B 1 - thiamine	• Vitamin A
• Vit B 2 - riboflavin	• Vitamin D
• Vit B 3 - niacin	• Vitamin E
• Vit B 5 – pantothenic acid	• Vitamin K
• Vit B 6 – pyridoxine	
• Vit B 6 – pyridoxal	
• Vit B 6 - pyridoxamine	
• Vit B 7 - biotin	
• Vit B 9 - folacin	
• Vit B12 - cobalamin	
• Vit C – ascorbic acid	

Table 3 – Water Soluble and Fat-Soluble Vitamins

Where are the two Vitamins B 4 and G?

As you scan the Table above you might be wondering why there is no Vitamin G or no Vitamin B 4. But as research progressed a number of chemicals originally identified as Vitamins have been re-classified.

- Riboflavin was originally classified as Vitamin G but has been re-classified as Vitamin B 2.
- Research subsequently revealed that the chemicals classified as Vitamins B 4, B 8, B 10 & B 11 could be synthesized by the body. They were therefore non-essential and no longer classified as Vitamins.

I come back to the point that the science backing up our understanding is work in progress and is rapidly evolving. Having said that, let's explore Vitamins D and K.

Essential Vitamins and another conundrum

Both Vitamins D and K present a similar conundrum to that of the Omega 3s, EPA and DHA.

It is true that the body can synthesize both these vitamins. But it is also true that our capacity to synthesize them varies considerably from one person to another.

For example, one factor in the synthesis of Vitamin D is exposure to sunlight. But what happens when a person only gets minimal exposure to sunlight on a regular basis?

Well, here in the UK it is estimated that across the whole population some 20-30% have low levels of Vitamin D. This is a significant issue.

The successful synthesis of Vitamin K in the Large Intestine is dependent on both other nutrients and possibly even the make-up of the Gut Flora as I will highlight in Chapter 17.

This begs the question "what other nutrients do we need to be including in our diet to facilitate the synthesis process?"

I prefer to treat them both as "Essential Nutrients" and make sure to get enough Vitamins D & K in my diet to complement any synthesized by my body.

Vitamin B12, Vitamin D and a Vegan Diet

Including both Vitamin B12 and Vitamin D can be a bit of a problem for vegans and strict vegetarians because most of the food sources are animal-based products.

Vitamin B12 also has a very particular characteristic. The body can only process small quantities at a time, so you must have a regular source in your daily diet. There is an open letter published on the Vegan Society website titled "What Every Vegan Should Know About Vitamin B12". **(Online Source 9).** The letter is very objective and provides sound advice on how to achieve this without animal-based products.

Vitamin D presents a rather different issue. The body can synthesize Vitamin D by exposing the skin to sunlight. However, there is a body of evidence suggesting many of us need to include it in our regular diet as well.

Natural sources of Vitamin D are animal based, with the exception of some mushrooms. However, synthetic Vitamin D can be produced from the plant sterol ergosterol. When added to foods such as milk, coconut milk or breakfast cereals these are referred to as "Fortified".

Vitamins and Fats

One big dilemma we face with Vitamins arises because some are water soluble, and others are fat soluble. So, with the relentless dietary advice to reduce or even eliminate dietary Fats…

…are we at risk of accidentally cutting out essential vitamins from our diet?

We'll tackle this a little further along our journey.

12. The Essential Minerals

The scientific research on our minerals seems to have gone hand in hand with research on the Vitamins. And as with the Vitamins, there are many great sources of information available. So, I won't try to replicate them here.

We use the term mineral in the context of our diet to describe a chemical element the body needs to perform necessary functions. All the minerals are Essential Nutrients, and they are listed in Table 4 below.

Macro or Major Minerals	Micro or Trace Minerals
• Calcium • Phosphorus • Magnesium • Sodium • Potassium • Chloride • Sulphur	• Iron • Manganese • Copper • Iodine • Zinc • Cobalt • Fluoride • Selenium • Molybdenum

Table 4 – Macro and Micro Minerals

And of course, there are a few peculiarities with the minerals. They are classified as Micronutrients in the overall diet and yet the minerals themselves are sub divided into:

- Macro or Major Minerals
- Micro or Trace Minerals

There are other peculiarities. For example, some sources include Molybdenum, but others don't. These peculiarities merely highlight that the science is catching up.

The list of Minerals in Table 4 is based on the list presented on the MyHealth.Alberta.ca website which also provides sample foods for the different minerals. **(Online Source 10).** And another great online source is the website for The Linus Pauling Institute at Oregon State University**. (Online Source 11).**

A great reference from the Linus Pauling Institute

I have included links to various online sources throughout these chapters on our Vitamins and Minerals. But if you want to read up in detail or have a reference to hand to dip into, I strongly recommend the online source published by Oregon State University **(Online Source 11 listed above**). The information is from the Linus Pauling Institute's Micronutrient Information Center on vitamins and minerals.

They also recommend Jane Higdon's book titled, *An Evidence-based Approach to Vitamins and Minerals: Health Benefits and Intake Recommendations.* **(Ref 6)** The book can be purchased from the Linus Pauling Institute, direct from Thieme Medical Publishers, or from your regular book sources.

Growing List of Nutrients

And finally, before you leave this Part of the Book just browse through all the Tables of the Amino Acids, Essential Fatty Acids, Vitamins and Minerals located throughout these Chapters.

Now we can really start to appreciate that the range of Amino Acids, Vitamins and Minerals we need on a regular basis is extensive. This highlights once again the need for a diversity of foods in our regular diet.

But this is only part of the story!

13. What about the Missing Food Types?

If you compare Table 1 at the start of Chapter 7 with Table 5 below, you may be wondering what happened to the other Food Types?

All Our 9 Food Types	Missing Food Types
Proteins	
Carbohydrates	Carbohydrates
Fats	
Water	
Minerals	
Vitamins	
Fibres	Fibres
Prebiotics & Probiotics	Prebiotics & Probiotics
Additional Micronutrients including Antioxidants, Phytochemicals & Enzymes	Additional Micronutrients including Antioxidants, Phytochemicals & Enzymes

Table 5 Missing Food Types

Back in Chapter 7 we covered how the Carbohydrates are not considered Essential Nutrients because the body can synthesize the Glucose it needs from all sorts of other foods, including other Sugars or Starches and from other Food Types namely from Fats and even from Proteins.

There are, however, a number of Food Types that cannot even be described in terms of being either Essential or Non-Essential.

Well, these Food Types are a little different because your body isn't digesting and absorbing them in the same way.

Rather, these nutrients are utilized by the body in a number of different ways. They are still vital to our overall nutrition.

As I found out how much they affected my own health I started calling them my **"Vital Nutrients"** and that is how I still refer to them.

So now we can move on to Part 3 where we explore our **Vital Nutrients**. And I have to say that this is the most exciting part of my diet and this Book.

Part 3 – The Missing Nutrients we need to know more about

14. The Nutrients I will call our Vital Nutrients

Now we turn our attention to the range of Food Types missing from our Essential and Non-Essential Nutrients.

Of the "7 Regular Food Types" referred to back in Chapter 6, the only Type not covered in the descriptions of Essential and Non-essential Nutrients is the Food Type – Fibres. The other missing Types are our Types 8 & 9 as shown in Table 6 below:

The Regular 7 Food Types	**Vital Nutrients**
Proteins	
Carbohydrates	
Fats	
Water	
Minerals	
Vitamins	
Fibres	Fibres
	Prebiotics & Probiotics
	Additional Micronutrients including Antioxidants, Phytochemicals & Enzymes

Table 6 The Missing Food Types are our Vital Nutrients

In fact, it might even seem odd that there are any Food Types we need in our diet that do not fall under the heading of either Essential or Non-Essential Nutrients. But I need to emphasize that they are treated differently because our body uses them in a slightly different way.

They are not digested and broken down into constituent parts for the body to use in the same way that, for example the proteins are broken down to amino acids which in turn are then used in cells or muscles.

These nutrients are ingested through our daily diet to **facilitate vital body functions,** so I started and continue to call them the **"Vital Nutrients".**

You will recall right at the start in the Introduction that I was trying to make sense of the beguilingly simple guideline:

- Eat 5 portions of Fruit & Veg a day.

Now we can delve a little deeper and explore how the Vital Nutrients in "Fruit & Veg" work with the body. **This is heavy going but hang in there because it is worth the effort!**

Why call them Vital Nutrients?

On my journey with Dr Younis, I started working on different ways to effectively re-boot my digestive system, especially my small intestine which had been ravaged by the tropical illness. Together we were working on two strategies:

1. Including plenty of fresh non-starchy vegetables plus modest portions of fruit as the preferred sources of fibres to aid digestion and absorption.

2. Testing ways to look after the Gut Flora or the Gut Microbiota.

Remember this was the early 1990s, research on the Gut Flora was not exactly mainstream. No matter, for the Gut Flora we tested two approaches:

- Including **probiotics** in my diet to boost levels of the "good bacteria", especially after using any antibiotics.
- Trying to simplify and test combinations of non-starchy vegetables to find what worked best for me.

It is fair to say that this approach was courting controversy. Dr Younis was sceptical about the standard dietary advice of that time which was to include loads of grain and seed fibre in the diet. I shared his scepticism.

I liked his holistic approach to medicine and health, so I deliberately started to include plenty of fresh non-starchy veg and fruits as my preferred source of fibres.

I still included grains, legumes and seeds in modest amounts and experimented with his various suggestions on probiotics.

Unfortunately, just as these strategies were starting to have a noticeable impact on my health, I lost contact with Dr Younis. I later found out he had tragically passed away. But I continued to use and refine the strategies, and I managed to regain a decent level of health again.

I maintained the strategies for some years and my health was fine with no major illnesses to speak of other than the odd cold. But over the years I let them slip.

Unfortunately, by 2013 and despite looking after everyone else, I was so lazy with my own diet that I had stopped using the strategies myself. As a result, my health was going backwards, and I was drifting into old age, at 55!

I was determined to turn this around to get my health and fitness back. So, I started to use and refine these same strategies all over again.

It was very noticeable that as soon as I started including my "5 a Day" of non-starchy veggies and fruit my health started improving.

And it was so easy to do that I was kicking myself for letting it go.

Anyway, through all this, these nutrients did not really fit into any recognized classification, so I just referred to the soluble fibres, insoluble fibres and probiotics as **my vital nutrients.**

Growing list of Vital Nutrients

New research coming into the public domain in recent years certainly seems to support some of the empirical observations I made on my own journey.

But interestingly, the list of vital nutrients was growing to now include:

- Insoluble Fibres
- Soluble Fibres
- Probiotics
- Prebiotics
- Additional Micronutrients including Antioxidants, Phytochemicals and Enzymes

The last of these I refer to as a single Type, but really it is really a "catch all" for nutrients that we are only just starting to understand. The Enzymes are beyond the scope of this book for now, but we come back to the Antioxidants and Phytochemicals shortly.

But you must bear with me. To really appreciate the role these Vital Nutrients play we first need to understand how the Digestive System works and the role of the different fibres.

15. The Digestive System and Daily Fiber Requirements

The Digestive System

The whole digestive system, also called the Gut or Gastrointestinal Tract, can be described in terms of the following three parts:

- Hollow organs including the mouth, pharynx, esophagus, stomach, small intestine, large intestine and anus. These organs are illustrated in **Fig 5** below.
- Solid organs including liver, pancreas and gallbladder.
- The Gut Flora, the part of our microbiome that resides in the digestive tract.

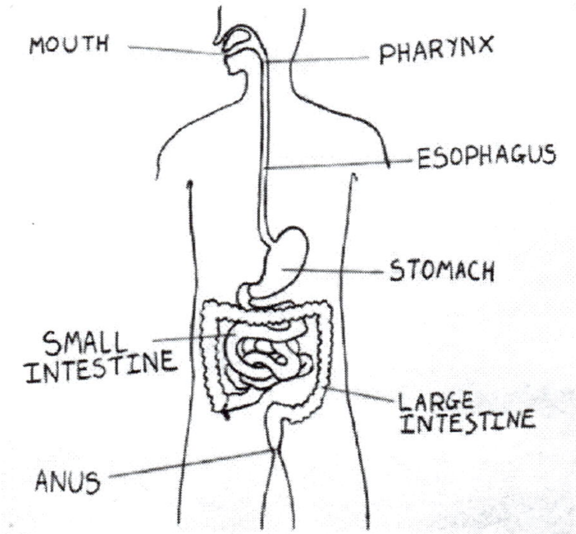

Fig 5. Hollow Organs of the Digestive System

Here we are particularly interested in the two Hollow Organs:

Small intestine – The duodenum is the first section of the small intestine, and this is where most of the digestion or breakdown of our food takes place. The digestive chemicals are secreted both within the small intestine and by the liver and pancreas.

The digestive chemicals include:

- The proteolytic enzymes, trypsin and chymotrypsin which combine with carboxypeptidase to breakdown the proteins.
- Pancreatic amylase that breaks down the carbohydrates
- Pancreatic Lipases that combine with the Bile Acids to breakdown the fats and digest fat soluble vitamins.

The following sections of the small intestine, the jejunum and the ilium are where much of this digested food is absorbed as it is mixed and churned by muscle action to bring it into contact with the villi lining the mucosa. The Gut Flora plays a key role in the absorption of the digested foods, and we will talk about that role in the following sections.

Large intestine – The large intestine is quite different in that no further digestive juices or enzymes are added here. However, the bacteria residing here as part of our Gut Flora play a key role by further breaking down the remaining nutrients. The Gut Flora also performs the vital function by converting some Vitamin K1 to Vitamin K2.

This organ is also where most of our vitamins, minerals and water are absorbed. And it seems that the soluble fibres play an important role facilitating the water absorption.

And we are also particularly interested in the:

Gut Flora – This is the part of the Human Microbiome that resides in the digestive tract.

We come back to these in the following sections but first we need to consider the recommended "Daily Intake of Fibre" as specified by notable sources such as the USDA and the University of California San Francisco.

Then we explore some of the functions the different Fibres perform and where we find them in our diet.

It will be very apparent that there are gaps between these functions and the wider health benefits, but we need to appreciate that the science is catching up fast.

A Problem with Recommended Daily Intake of Fibre

The health benefits of fibre in your regular diet are now widely reported. For example, a summary online article titled "Should I be eating more fiber?" by Katherine McManus published by the Harvard Medical School, **(Online Source 12).**

The article highlights how suitable levels of our different Fibres can:

- Help lower bad cholesterol levels.

and decrease the risk of dying from conditions including:

- Heart Disease
- Cancer
- Stroke
- Type 2 Diabetes

Who would not want these health benefits? But exactly how some of these health benefits come about is still work in progress. Even so, the article reports that the USDA recommends a daily amount of Fibres for adults up to the age of 50 as follows:

25 grams for women

38 grams for men

The recommendations for adults over the age of 50 are:

21 grams for women

30 grams for men

Yet on average, the article goes on to say, these same American adults **eat just 10-15 grams a day**! And I suspect the same is true here in the UK.

If the health benefits of dietary fibres are so well known, how is it that so many people still eat too little?

Maybe it is because many of us don't know about both Soluble and Insoluble Fibres. Or maybe it's because we don't know how to actually measure out 25/38 grams of fibre in our regular food?

Or is it because it is just difficult to understand how fibres can have such a profound impact on our health.

After all, how do dietary fibres help reduce the risk of Heart Disease or Cancer?

Part of this confusion is that the fibres are not digested and absorbed like proteins, fats or carbs. They are ingested through our daily diet to **facilitate vital body functions.**

So, what are these vital body functions?

To understand how the fibres facilitate these vital functions, we must firstly investigate three aspects of our Digestive System. We will tackle them in this order:

1. Small Intestine
2. Gut Flora
3. Large Intestine

We start by exploring the physical attributes of the Small Intestine.

16. The Small Intestine & our Fibers

The importance of the small intestine in both our diet and our overall health now receives a lot of attention because it is here that much of our food is digested and absorbed. However, it seems that much of the modern research focusses on the role of the gut flora that resides here. We will come back to the Gut Flora in the following Chapter.

But first we begin by exploring the combination of one particular physical attribute of this organ and the roles our vital nutrients play in conjunction with this attribute. The combination makes this an astonishing organ.

Physical Attributes of the Small Intestine

The small intestine appears to be a simple tubular organ neatly folded in the space between our stomach and our pelvis. However, the simple appearance is deceptive.

In an average adult this tubular organ measures just an inch (2.5 cm) in diameter when non-dilated or empty of food. This can expand to an inch and a half (4 cm) when dilated. The length varies depending on age but for most adults it will measure some 18-24 feet (5.4 – 7.3 m) in length.

The innermost layer of this tubular structure is a folded membrane called the Small Intestinal Mucosa, Mucosa for short, which surrounds the open space within the tube, called the Lumen. This folded Mucosa is astonishing.

In the average adult the small intestine would be some 20 feet or 6m long. If the Mucosa was unfolded and laid out flat, it would have a height of some 16 feet or 5m. This gives a surface area of some 320 square feet or 30 square metres. Laid flat this would nearly cover a ¼ of a tennis court. Held vertically it would be nearly as high as a small house as illustrated in **Fig 6** below.

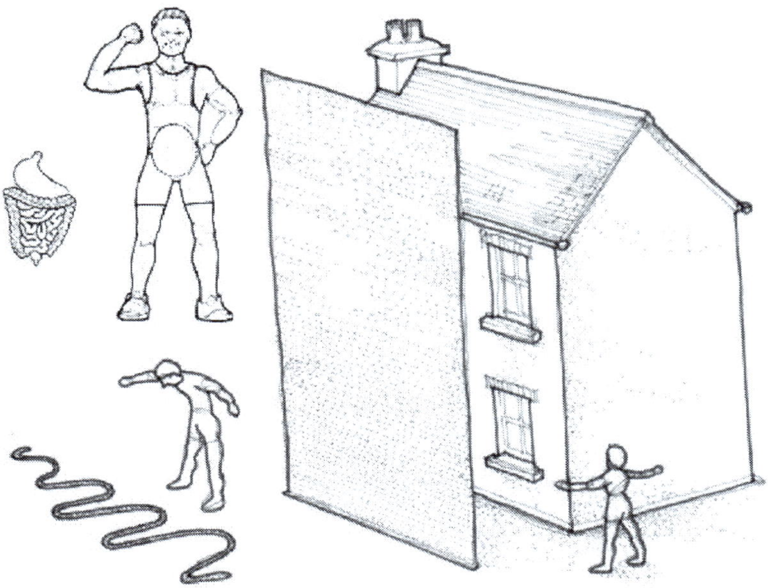

Fig 6. The astonishing scale of the Mucosa

However, the Mucosa is not only folded but also covered in finger like projections called villi which increase the surface area again. Some sources estimate a fourfold increase in surface area.

So, the total surface area of the small intestinal mucosa in the average adult is close to the size of the whole tennis court. This vast surface area is home to a significant portion of our Gut Flora.

But here we are interested in the physical environment created by folding and packing the vast mucosa into a tube a mere inch or 2.5 cm in diameter.

All the food we eat must pass through this tiny, densely packed tube, squeezing through the small spaces between all the tight folds of the Mucosa.

What purpose does this vast surface area serve?

As food passes through the small intestine the combination of the tiny, intricate pathways created by the folded mucosa and the muscular action of the organ walls:

- Churns the partially digested food enabling efficient mixing with the new digestive juices released here. The digestion or breakdown of the proteins and carbs continues, and the breakdown of the fats begins.

- The churning action then brings the digested, or broken down, amino acids, carbs and fats into direct contact with the Mucosa and the gut flora residing on that vast surface enabling absorption of nutrients to take place.

Now that we can visualize the structure of this organ, we can start to appreciate just how important it is that the largely solid food that enters the mouth is fully prepared to pass through this small tube hosting the vast, tightly folded membrane. The consistency of the food at this point is vital to enable efficient digestion and absorption to take place.

Let's take a step back and consider how the food we have eaten is prepared for this journey.

Preparing food to pass through the Small Intestine

The digestion process begins in the mouth where the chewing action starts the physical process of breaking down the food. This action also stimulates the production of saliva which contains several enzymes including amylase, lysozyme and lingual lipase.

This mix of food and saliva passes down the esophagus and into the stomach where a combination of pepsinogen, which converts to pepsin, and lipase continue to break down the foods.

This combination of food and enzymes passing from the stomach into the first section of the small intestine, the duodenum, is mixed into **a malleable paste called chyme**.

But now that we are aware of the physical constraints of the Small Intestine, we can appreciate an often-overlooked factor.

The consistency of the chyme plays an important role determining how efficiently it passes through the surprisingly complex physical structure of the small intestine. This in turn has a significant impact on the efficiency of the digestion and absorption of the nutrients.

What does the science tell us?

Most sources describe the chyme just in terms of the partially digested foods combined with the various digestive juices secreted from the different glands and added to the mix along the way. This all creates a malleable paste or semi fluid mass.

But more and more sources, like the University of California, San Francisco in an article titled "Increasing Fiber Intake" published on their website UCSF Health, **(Online Source 13)** now highlight the role of the soluble and insoluble fibres. Their roles can be summarized as follows:

- Insoluble fibres are not broken down by the digestion process, they remain largely intact and help bind the chyme.
- Soluble fibres absorb water to produce a soft gooey paste that helps suspend the smaller particles of digested or broken-down pieces of food.

Now that we understand the physical space the chyme passes through in the small intestine, we can appreciate how the Soluble Fibres help separate and suspend the broken-down particles of food.

Then the Insoluble Fibres help bind and mix the food particles with the digestive juices as the muscle action churns the whole lot through the length of the organ. The combined effect also helps to bring more digested food into close contact with the Gut Flora sitting on the mucosa to aid absorption.

It does seem that the combination of insoluble and soluble fibres plays a vital role creating the ideal consistency of soft malleable paste required for the chyme to pass through the small intestine.

This ideal consistency allows efficient digestion and absorption of the nutrients.

Searching for these Soluble and Insoluble Fibres?

As I was searching for the best sources of Soluble and Insoluble Fibres I kept coming up against what seemed to be the standard advice, namely:

- The best sources of fibres were grains, cereals and seeds.
- The soluble fibres didn't really rate a mention.

This took me back to my discussions with Dr Younis and the scepticism about the advice to eat so much grain and seeds.

I had already found that the non-starchy vegetables and fruits seemed to work very effectively for me, and I was curious to know why. I started to look at my vegetables and fruit in a new way as I set out to get the absolute most from my "5 a Day".

A New Dimension to Fibres

But now my journey coincided with the emergence of new science on our Gut Flora.

The new research seemed to support the basic understanding I had about the Probiotics and directly including good microbes in my diet.

The research also identified a new Food Type, the Prebiotics. Well, new to me. This raised two questions:

1. What is the difference between Probiotics and Prebiotics?
2. And how are Prebiotics related to Fibres?

Just as I thought I was getting to grips with how my digestive system worked, the new research on the Human Microbiome opened up a range of new issues and options.

17. Gut Flora, our Second Brain and Probiotics & Prebiotics

Microbiome, Microbiota and our Gut Flora

Evidence of microorganisms in the normal human system was first identified in the mid-1880s by the Austrian paediatrician Theodore Escherich. But it is only as recently as 1986 that the Gut-Brain Axis was first demonstrated in groundbreaking research by Linda R Hegstrand and Roberta Jean Hine, *see below.

The origins of the now widely recognized concepts of the "Microbiota" and "Human Microbiome" are unclear but in her paper "History of Medicine: Origin of the term microbiome and why it matters" in the Human Microbiome Journal ***(Online Source 14)**, Susan Prescott highlights the role of different researchers who deserve much of the credit.

One thing is clear, by the mid-1990s, the term Human Microbiome became mainstream.

In 2007 the National Human Genome Research Institute (NHGRI) sponsored the Human Microbiome Project (HMP). This project funded 5 years of co-ordinated research conducted by a consortium of nearly 80 universities and scientific institutes around the world.

This is cutting edge scientific research that still continues at a rapid pace. In fact, research results from the HMP are completely redefining our understanding of the human condition.

So, what is the Microbiome?

The Microbiome is the name given to **all the microbes** that live both on and in the whole human body. It is the collection of all the microbes, including bacteria, fungi, protozoa and viruses. For the average adult the microbiome is made up of some 75-200 trillion microbes.

Staggeringly that is 2-4x the number of cells in the body.

But that is only half the story because this will be made up of a vast diversity of strains of all the different microbes. There are over 4000 different strains of bacteria alone.

This collection of microbes is not spread evenly around the body. Different parts of this whole Microbiome reside in or on different locations or areas of the body and these are referred to as our different Microbiota.

The collection of microbes residing in the Digestive System are therefore known collectively as the Gut Microbiota and are also often referred to as our Gut Flora.

Elizabeth Thursby and Nathalie Juge present an excellent summary in their paper titled "Introduction to the human gut microbiota" published online in the Biochemical Journal, **(Online Source 15**).

A delicate Balancing Act

We will refer to the diversity of strains of microbes including bacteria, fungi, protozoa and viruses of the Microbiome as the whole spectrum. Each different microbiota may contain just a portion of this spectrum, their own mini spectrum. So, the Gut Microbiota contains it's own mini spectrum.

Within the whole spectrum there are "good" microbes, like beneficial bacteria and "bad" microbes, also referred to as pathogens. Likewise, the mini spectra in all the different Microbiota also have a mix of "good" and "bad" microbes.

Indeed, it seems that the vast population of microbes is in a constant state of flux and **this delicate balancing act is an essential part of the human condition**.

This delicate balancing act is going on in all the mini spectra of all the different microbiota. In a simplistic analogy, we can infer that when the balance is about right, we are healthy and when it tips away from this, we can become less healthy.

A Unique Signature and an exciting Breakthrough

Before we go any further, we need to understand that there is no one standard make-up of the whole microbiome or one standard make-up for any of the different microbiota that every human should fit into.

We are all different. We each have a **unique microbiome** and **unique gut flora.** The variation from one individual to another can depend on a host of factors. These variations can be modest or significant. As such, our individual Microbiome is a bit like **a signature**.

The one constant for all of us though, is the delicate balance between the "good" and "bad" microbes. And this leads us to one really exciting breakthrough from all the research.

We can all influence a balance that promotes good health, and we can do this with our diet.

It is interesting to note that even back in the mid-19th century the French scientist, Antoine Béchamps was suggesting a link and even a dependency between the health of humans and the bacteria that were present in the body, and he compared this collection of Bacteria to something like an eco-system. In his wonderful book *"Till the cows come home"* **(Ref 7),** Philip Walling talks about these ideas and how Béchamp put forward the idea that good health was in part a function of the balance in this system.

Modern research on the microbiome confirms this idea of an ecosystem in a delicate state of balance and to understand why this is so important we need to explore what our Gut Flora does for us.

What our Gut Flora does for us

We are particularly interested in the roles our Gut Flora plays in the two hollow organs of the digestive tract:

> **Gut Flora in the Small Intestine** – Here the Flora would seem to be dispersed across the vast surface area of the small intestinal mucosa described in Chapter 16. Some sources regard the Flora as even forming part of the **intestinal mucosal barrier.**

This barrier effectively enables the passage of small particles of nutrients into the bloodstream whilst blocking the passage of unwanted larger particles and microorganisms.

Although numerically numerous, the Flora here shows a modest diversity by all accounts. However, the Flora does seem to perform or enable several vital functions. These include aiding the digestion of Folic Acid and Vitamin K1. The Flora also helps stimulate the production of IL8 or Interleukin 8 and as such the Gut Flora can even be described as a gland.

Gut Flora in the Large Intestine – Whilst this organ is a simpler tubular structure compared to the small intestine, the Flora are more diverse and complicated.

The Flora are vital to digestion as they break down some of the Insoluble Fibres by fermentation to produce fatty acids that the body can then absorb as a nutrient. This fermentation process is also critical to the production of Vitamin K2. This process also stimulates the production of Vitamin B7, Biotin.

These are simplified descriptions of the role of the Flora in the two organs. A more complete description is far more complicated and beyond the scope of this book. But these examples do illustrate the **symbiotic relationship** between the **Human Microbiome** and the **Human Body**.

It seems that there is an interdependency. The Human Body needs the Microbiome to enable or specifically perform Vital Functions. In the case of the Small Intestine, this symbiotic relationship goes further still.

Gut Flora, the Small Intestine and Our Second Brain

The symbiotic relationship between the small intestines and the Gut Flora is so remarkable that it:

- Controls the digestion and absorption of food.
- Impacts on the immune system.
- Communicates directly with the brain to control or at least impact on our sense of hunger and/or satiation.

- Communicates directly with the brain to control or at least impact on cognitive abilities such as memory and senses including emotions.

In fact, the combination of the structure of this impressive organ and wider impact of the Gut Flora on our immune system and the brain leads some people to refer to the combination of our small intestine and the resident microbiota as:

Our second brain

There are many sources exploring the links between our gut flora, the food we eat and human behaviour. One excellent source is *"Gut well soon"* by the integrative health therapist Catherine Rogers **(Ref 8)**. This is an exciting area of research.

How can we control the balance of Good and Bad Microbes?

The whole Human Microbiome, including the Gut Flora, is made up of living organisms.

The whole range of different microbes, be they bacteria, fungi, protozoa or viruses, are all living organisms so they reproduce, and they can die. And as living organisms they also feed.

So, the idea that the Gut Flora is in a delicate state of balance between Good and Bad microbes raises the question:

How can we increase the population size of the good microbes relative to the bad microbes, tipping the balance in favour of better health?

In other words, can we increase the population size of the good microbes by:

- Directly digesting more of the good microbes in the food we eat
- Preferentially feeding the good microbes already in the Gut Flora so that they flourish at the expense of the bad microbes.

Which brings us to the two Vital Food Types:

- **Probiotics** – These are foods we eat that contain the good microbes.

- **Prebiotics** – These are food we eat that our good microbes feed on.

And conversely, can we inadvertently increase the population size of the bad microbes by eating:

- **Bad Prebiotics** – These are foods that preferentially feed the bad microbes so that they flourish at the expense of the good microbes.

Searching for our Probiotics and Prebiotics

The Probiotics and Prebiotics are one of the most exciting areas of our diet. But just like the Fibres, they are not easy to categorize and list.

What we can say at this stage is that as specific nutrient Types they occur in a range of foods, and some are closely associated with the different fibres. But before we go into more detail about where to find them, we need to explore our Antioxidants and Phytochemicals.

18. The Lymphatic System, Free Radicals, Antioxidants & Phytochemicals

Both the Lymphatic System and the Antioxidants are rather misunderstood. They deserve a lot more of our attention because they both play key roles in removing waste from the body. We start with the Lymphatic system.

The Lymphatic System

Much like the cardiovascular system, this is a network of vessels, or tubes, that reaches all the muscles, every organ and every cell of the body. This system also includes the Lymph Nodes, spleen, thymus, ducts and tonsils.

These vessels are not quite as well defined as the more familiar arteries and veins of the cardiovascular system, but they still reach every cell in the body. There are two characteristics to note:

- The Lymphatic System **DOES NOT** have a pumping organ like the heart. This system is pumped by deep diaphragm breathing from strenuous activity, specific breathing exercises and even massaging.
- The Lymphatic System can carry up to **6-7 times the volume** of liquid carried in the cardiovascular system when fully utilized.

While the primary role of the cardiovascular system is to distribute nutrients around the body, the equivalent primary role of the lymphatic system is to remove waste products like the free radicals from the muscles and cells.

Free Radicals

But what exactly are Free Radicals? An old article on the online publication Medical News Today provided an elegant description:

> *Free radicals are waste substances produced by the cells as the body processes food and reacts to the environment. If the body cannot process and remove free radicals efficiently, oxidative stress can result. This can harm cells and body function. Free radicals are also known as reactive oxygen species (ROS).*

The same article went on to highlight the growing evidence of a link between this state of oxidative stress and a range of illnesses including:

- Heart disease
- Cancer
- Arthritis
- Stroke
- Respiratory diseases
- Immune deficiency and more

Whilst that article does not seem to be live anymore, they still have two relevant articles, **(Online Source 16)**.

The first article is titled "How do free radicals affect the body?" and is reviewed by Rose Wilson and Zawn Villines. The second article is titled "How does oxidative stress affect the body?" and is reviewed by Stacy Sampson and Jamie Eske.

And it is good to note that the link between a fully functional Lymphatic System Free Radicals and good health is finally getting the attention it deserves.

Another excellent source of information is the website and blog for Dr Jennifer Weinberg. Her article titled "Revitalize Your Lymphatic System for Clearer Skin, Vibrant Energy & More Efficient Metabolism", is a great place to start, **(Online Source 17**).

Searching for our Antioxidants and Phytochemicals

To remove the unwanted free radicals, the body produces Antioxidants. These are endogenous antioxidants.

We can also include other Antioxidants in our diet, and these are the exogenous Antioxidants. It is the second group that we are covering here.

As with the Fibres, Probiotics and Prebiotics I would like to present a list or table of Antioxidants along the lines of the Essential Vitamins for example. But that doesn't quite work for the Antioxidants either, but for a different reason.

Rather than any individual nutrient being an Antioxidant, it seems more appropriate to describe various nutrients as having "Antioxidant Properties".

So, for example, some Vitamins and Minerals have antioxidant properties including:

The Vitamins A, C & E

The Minerals Manganese (Mn), & Selenium (Se)

But in addition to these minerals and vitamins, research has identified another group of compounds that occur in fresh plant foods that appear to offer health benefits. These are the Phytochemicals.

These are three major groups of Phytochemicals and within these there are four main "families or groups of similar compounds" with strong antioxidant properties, as follows:

1. Carotenoids like Lycopene (Red) & Lutein (Green)
2. Flavonoids like resveratrol & hesperidin (vivid colours)
3. Ellagic Acid found in many berries.
4. Allium Compounds

These are described in an excellent article on the types of phytochemicals originally published online by Emilia Klapp on the original "Sharecare" website. The article also provided a useful overview of food sources for these phytochemicals which I will refer to again in the following Chapter. **(Online Source 18).**

The Lymphatic System and our Antioxidants

There seems to be a growing body of research indicating that a combination of a fully functioning Lymphatic system and a healthy selection of Antioxidants can help remove the unwanted free radicals from our bodies. This is an interesting and relatively new area of research and science is rapidly catching up.

More to Discover about our Phytochemicals

It seems that our Antioxidants are just some of the chemicals described as Phytochemicals or Phytonutrients. But what are the extra chemicals?

The first thing to bear in mind is that the term "Phytochemicals" literally means chemicals found in plants and this covers a huge range of chemicals. They often give the bright colours to plants such as the Blue in Blueberries and Orange in Carrots.

I have already mentioned three major groups of Phytochemicals where we find chemicals with strong antioxidant properties. But there are now considered to be anywhere between five, seven or even twelve main groups of Phytochemicals depending on which source you use.

This might seem odd, but we must remember that this area of nutrition research is very much in its infancy. If we start with the Groups listed by The National Library of Medicine, **(Online Source 19),** they list seven as follows:

- Carotenoids
- Indoles
- Glucosinolates
- Organosulfur Compounds
- Phytosterols
- Polyphenols
- Saponins

Other sources refer to up to twelve "Major Classifications" and may also include:

- Polysaccharides
- Lectins
- Terpenes
- Alkaloids
- Polyacetylenes
- Chlorophyll
- Dietary Fibres

Even then, in the paper titled "Clinical Evidence of the Benefits of Phytonutrients in Human Healthcare" the authors refer to specific chemicals that many of us will be familiar with and these include:

- Flavonoids
- Caffeine
- Tannins

Some of these Phytochemicals have "Antioxidant Properties". And it seems that this is the nature of these chemicals. Other Phytochemicals seem to have properties that aid or facilitate other specific functions or properties including:

- Anticancer
- Anti-inflammatory
- Antiviral
- Improved cognitive function

It is also important to note that some Phytochemicals such as Lectins can be harmful to our health. For example, Kidney Beans contain the Lectin Phytohaemagglutinin, which is a naturally occurring toxin. For the beans to be edible they must first be allowed to soak in water and then be cooked by boiling for sufficient time. Other Lectins may also be removed from foods in a similar way.

Furthermore, some Polyphenols and Tannins act as inhibitors preventing the digestion of different minerals or vitamins from some of the fruit and veg we might eat. And they may even prevent the digestion of vitamins or minerals from other foods we might eat with our fruit and veg. So true to form our nutrition is always rather nuanced.

Even so, this shouldn't distract us from the ever-growing list of positive benefits because it does seem that more and more functions and health benefits are being identified.

But perhaps most significantly there seems to be a growing body of research indicating that the real health value of the Phytochemicals is in the combination of many individual nutrients working together. And I will come back to this again in Chapter 20.

19. Where do we find our Vital Nutrients?

It seems that our Vital Nutrients are important, but they are really quite messy to deal with. We can't list the individual nutrients, nor can we measure them out precisely either.

We need to explore in detail where we find them in our diet. This in turn will highlight just how important the "5 a day" rule is and how we can all adapt and fine tune this rule around our own lifestyle. We start with our Fibres.

Where do we find the Soluble and Insoluble Fibres?

There is a growing body of research available on the best sources of soluble and insoluble fibres. I will refer again to the information article produced by the University of California, San Francisco for educational purposes only. **(Online Source 13)**

The article lists the key sources of fibres as follows:

1. Grains & Cereals
2. Legumes & Beans
3. Fruits & Vegetables
4. Fibre Supplements

This article puts a lot of emphasis on "Grains & Cereals". In fact, the notes under that first heading go on to say:

- As a general rule, include at least one serving of whole grain in every meal.

I might not particularly agree with that, but I'm very happy with the first item under the third heading, "Fruits & Vegetables" which is:

- Eat at least five servings of fruits and vegetables each day. Fresh fruit is slightly higher in fiber than canned. Eat the peel whenever possible - it's easier than peeling or eating around it.

This also leads me back to the advice offered by Dr Younis all those years ago. He was sceptical about the high levels of grain recommended back in the 1990s. He felt the non-starchy vegetables and fruits were the best sources of the fibres we all need and that grains should be eaten in moderation primarily as an energy food.

Back then I did include grains, starchy vegetables, legumes and beans in my diet and still do. But I treat them primarily as sources of Carbohydrate. And as such, their Fibre content complemented the Fibre intake from my modified **"5 a day" rule** which includes:

- Generous portions of non-starchy vegetables either cooked or served as salads to make up 4 of my "5 a day".

  COMBINED WITH

- Moderate fruit portions to make up the fifth.

As you read on through the Chapters in this Part of the Book you will see that many of the fresh non-starchy vegetables and fruits are also sources for other Vital Nutrients, especially prebiotics and antioxidants. And of course, these same plant foods are important sources of vitamins and minerals.

I quickly came to appreciate that these were the stars of my diet, and I elaborate on this aspect in the following Chapters.

Why do we eat so little Fibre?

This all seems reasonable enough and yet as I pointed out in Chapter 15, despite this information being widely available American adults eat just 10-15 grams of fibre a day which is well below the recommended levels. I was the same and I don't know why.

My own experience all those years ago indicated that I too was eating far too little Fibre of any sort. Introducing them into my diet made a huge impact. So much so that I was finally able to say goodbye to living on pills and shakes. However, a few years later I foolishly let my eating habits slip away again.

But as soon as I started following my **modified "5 a day" rule** again the benefits to my health were quickly apparent. In just a few months I was able to turn my health around and get back on track. But now I really was just getting started! Understanding my Gut Flora would change things again!

Where do we find our Probiotics?

Back in Chapter 17 we covered how we can theoretically boost the population of good microbes in our Gut Flora by including them in our diet.

The foods and drinks that contain these live good bacteria or other good microbes are called our Probiotics. They are produced by fermentation and by a quirk of human ingenuity we humans have developed various fermentation processes to prepare and store food. Three key sources include:

Dairy Based

- Live yoghurt, including Lactobacillus bulgaricus and Streptococcus thermophilus.
- Kefir, a type of fermented milk drink

Vegetable Based

- Kimchi, a type of fermented vegetables originating in Korea
- Fermented vegetables such as Pickles and Sauerkraut

Legume Based

- Tempeh, a type of fermented Soy product from Indonesia
- Miso, a paste made from fermented soy from Japan that may also include barley or rice

More recently an additional variation has been introduced:

Cultured Probiotics

- Gut friendly microbes such as Lactobacillus Acidophilus are prepared in tablet or other supplement forms.

The use of Cultured Lactobacillus Acidophilus added to Live Yoghurt to counteract the effects of antibiotics became an accepted practice here in the UK back in the 1990s and continues to be so today. But every source I have read recommends that cultured probiotics in this form should only be taken on the advice of medical professionals.

We Have Been Eating Fermented Foods for Thousands of Years

There are all sorts of foods from around the world prepared by fermenting. So, as we start to appreciate the role of our Probiotics it might come as a surprise to note that there are already all sorts of foods that actually fit into this Food Type. You probably include some in your diet already!

These are not new foods. In fact, we humans have been eating all sorts of fermented foods for thousands of years and enjoying the benefits. This is an important point that I will come back to again shortly.

Jillian Levy presents a list of fermented foods in her article titled Fermented Foods for a Healthy Gut and Overall Health published online **(Online Source 20)**. And for some of us the list of fermented foods may be growing. For example, in addition to the specific foods listed above an unexpected item like sourdough bread is made by fermenting the dough and is becoming more popular, well certainly here in the UK.

Unfortunately, there is a possible downside. Much as I like various pickled vegetables like onions and gherkins, some modern pickling processes do not retain the live Probiotic content. Sometimes so-called progress can be so frustrating.

But on the bright side, I do happen to like Live Yoghurt and include this quite regularly. So, I am quite happy that I'm including regular portions of Probiotics in my diet.

Where do we find our Prebiotics?

In Chapter 17 we described how the Gut Flora is made up of living organisms and these living organisms need to feed.

In other words, some of the food we eat is feeding the microbes of our Gut Flora. This raises two interesting questions:

1. Can we preferentially feed the good microbes to maintain a healthy balance?
2. Do some of the foods we eat promote the bad microbes in our Gut Flora?

The term Prebiotics is used for the nutrients that feed the good microbes of the Gut Flora, and these Prebiotics include a range of both soluble and insoluble fibres. So, it seems that role of each of the Types of fibre can be twofold:

- Some soluble fibres perform a key function in the creation of chyme and are also key nutrients for some of our good microbes.
- Some insoluble fibres help to bind and mix the chyme as it passes through the small intestine and then feed our good microbes in the large intestine. The resulting short chain fatty acids can then be absorbed and used as a nutrient by the body.

We must remember, this is all very new. There seems to be a growing body of evidence that including a wide range of soluble and insoluble fibres in the diet will provide a range of nutrients for our good microbes.

There is no definitive list but there are now many sources providing useful lists for quick reference.

I will refer to the list of 19 Foods suggested in the article by Arlene Semeco and Erin Kelly published online by Healthline **(Online Source 21)**. Their list is reproduced in Table 7 on the following page.

Now this list might look daunting at first, I mean how many people have Yacon Root or Seaweed sitting in their kitchen right now.

But actually, if you take a closer look, it is quite possible that you already include some of the other foods on the list in your regular diet. Adding a few more won't really take that much effort.

• Chicory Root	• Apples
• Dandelion Greens	• Konjac Root
• Jerusalem Artichokes	• Cocoa
• Garlic	• Burdock Roots
• Onions	• Flaxseed
• Leeks	• Yacon Root
• Asparagus	• Jicama Root
• Bananas	• Wheat Bran
• Barley	• Seaweed
• Oats	

Table 7 Good Prebiotics

From the article by Arlene Semeco and Erin Kelly published online by Healthline.

So, what about the foods that promote our bad microbes? Perhaps we should call these our Bad Prebiotics.

Where do we find our Bad Prebiotics?

For the Bad Prebiotics I will refer to the Newsletter of the online publication Medical News Today. The article was written by Zawn Villines and reviewed by Hope Warshaw. **(Online Source 22**).

The article highlights a classification into four types of food, as opposed to our Food Types. We'll scan three of these and cover the fourth in more detail. Starting with:

> **Animal Proteins –** The Newsletter notes "There is some research suggesting that diets high in protein and particularly

animal proteins can disrupt the gut flora promoting the bad microbes."

But we have already discussed how our true protein requirements are in fact quite modest. This may be just one of the possible negative effects of eating too much protein.

Foods containing antibiotics – Residual antibiotics in our food chain can disrupt our Gut Flora in the same way as antibiotic medication. This highlights a problem with the widespread use of antibiotics in many areas of less ethical mass livestock production.

Fried Foods – There is some research suggesting that Fried foods, especially when using saturated fats and trans fats can act as bad prebiotics preferentially feeding the bad microbes.

The fourth category is referred to as **High FODMAP Foods.** This term is derived from a number of carb foods that may cause digestive issues, and the name is derived from:

Fermentable **O**ligo, **D**i, **M**ono-saccharides **A**nd **P**olyols

So what are the High FODMAP Foods?

High FODMAP Foods – This fourth type includes:

- Processed foods containing high fructose corn syrup, sorbitol and other artificial sweeteners.
- Fruit juices
- Agave, honey, and many other sweeteners
- Condiments such as jam, relish, and hummus

Comparing the Good Prebiotics with the Bad does highlight how eating fresh recognizable foods seems to be a good indicator of health benefits.

This does not mean we should avoid foods such as fruit juices, honey or agave altogether, rather it highlights that we should treat these foods with some caution and only eat them in moderation.

Reviewing our Probiotics, Prebiotics and Bad Prebiotics

This is all really quite messy. We have some foods that we can ingest that have potential to provide more good microbes for our Gut Flora and some foods that may preferentially feed the good microbes already present in our Gut Flora.

But we also have foods that have the potential to disrupt those benefits by preferentially feeding our bad microbes.

We talked about how our Gut Flora impacts not just on our digestion but on our overall health. The impact of processed foods, lifestyle and other factors is described by S Bengmark **(Online Source 23)** as follows:

1. Lund University, Ideon Research Centre, Suite 230, Beta Building, S22370 Lund, Sweden

From the Paper Titled - The "new" lifestyle—a threat to health?

> *It is increasingly evident that human diseases are most often related to lifestyle, and should in theory be preventable. The stress of modern life, our reduced physical activity, and our consumption of manipulated and processed foods, and of chemicals—including pharmaceuticals—all contribute to our decreasing resistance to disease.*

He goes on the say:

> *Perhaps even more important than the decrease in these food ingredients, is the fact that prehistoric food contained several thousand times more bacteria, mainly the so called probiotic bacteria. Prehistoric methods of food preservation were either drying, or, more commonly, storing in holes dug into the ground, where the food became naturally fermented. This is how Stone Age man learned to produce most of our still common fermented foods, such as beer, wine, green olives, and sauerkraut. Our modern lifestyle has dramatically reduced the availability of foods produced by natural fermentation.*

It seems that we humans may have adapted to fermented foods over thousands and even hundreds of thousands of years. But modern foods, eating styles and lifestyles may be inadvertently undoing all that good. This is a topic we will pick up again in the next Chapter.

But this idea of Good and Bad Prebiotics also highlights the issue of how the body needs to clean out the unwanted and unhealthy parts of our diet as well as the natural waste products.

And this is where the Antioxidants come in.

Where do we find the Antioxidants and other Phytochemicals?

In the previous Chapter we covered the four main "families or groups" of phytochemicals with strong antioxidant properties. and referred to the excellent article published online by Emilia Klapp on the original "Sharecare" website, **(Online Source 18)** Here we list four main "families" again as follows:

1. **Carotenoids** like Lycopene (Red) & Lutein (Green) – apricot, mangoes, papaya, red peppers, tomatoes,

2. **Flavonoids** like resveratrol & hesperidin (vivid colours) – apples, cherries,

3. **Ellagic Acid** found in many berries.

4. **Allium Compounds** – the main sources are sometimes referred to as the allium vegetables. These are the richest source of organosulfur compounds in the human diet and with the richest of the lot being garlic.

The short list above also highlights how Phytochemicals often provide the colours and especially the vivid colours across many fruits and vegetables.

Emilia Klapp's expanded list shown in Table 8 on the following page, highlights additional health benefits over and above the Antioxidant properties.

Building a case for the "5 a Day" Rule

As we scan through all the Vital Nutrients, we can see they can be found in a range of different foods. But interestingly many of them are particularly abundant in the non-starchy vegetables and fruits.

- **Carotenoids** such as beta-carotene, lycopene, and lutein protect fat cells, blood, and other bodily fluids from free radicals. They can be found in apricots, mangoes, papayas, watermelon, spinach, sweet potatoes, corn, red peppers, romaine lettuce, and tomatoes, to name a few sources.
- **Flavonoids** such as resveratrol, hesperidin, anthocyanin, quercetin, and tangeritin act against inflammation and prevent platelets from sticking together. They also block the enzymes that raise blood pressure. They can be found in vitamin-C-rich foods such as apples, cherries, blueberries, grapefruit, oranges, plums, strawberries, broccoli, and kale.
- **Ellagic acid** decreases cholesterol levels and is found in strawberries, blackberries, blueberries, kiwifruit, raspberries, currants, and red grapes. Strawberries especially have been found in studies to inhibit certain enzymes, reducing the inflammation process in the arteries.
- **Allium compounds** protect the cardiovascular and immune systems. They are found in onions, scallions, leeks, chives, and garlic.

Table 8 Food Sources for Antioxidants

But the vital nutrients are not as clearly or easily identified as our other nutrients. They seem often to be properties attributed to families or groups of chemicals too numerous or vast to present in a simple table form like our Minerals or Vitamins for example. And yet surprisingly, it seems to be that the real health value of Phytochemicals is in the combination of many individual nutrients working together.

It seems that we are continuing to build the case to embrace the "5 a Day" Rule, so let's explore that in a bit more detail.

20 Cutting edge science and the "5 a Day" Rule

Working through the previous Chapters you can be forgiven for thinking that the classification of our Vital Nutrients is quite vague compared to our Vitamins, Minerals and Amino Acids. Even just trying to classify our Vital Nutrients into any sort of easy list is a messy process, but part of that is because the science on our Vital Nutrients really is so very new.

Much of our understanding of Probiotics and Prebiotics, for example, only emerged from the Human Microbiome Project which ran 2007-2012. It turns out that some of the foods that we humans have been eating for thousands of years just happen to contain these nutrients. So, we just need to start including them back in our diet again.

Phytochemicals are even less well defined, but they do seem to offer a range of health benefits. For example, "families of similar compounds" found in the fresh plant foods we eat appear to act as Antioxidants. These "families" include both flavonoids and other phytochemicals.

But rather than trying to classify some of the Phytochemicals as Antioxidants, perhaps it is more accurate to say that some of these Phytochemicals have "Antioxidant Properties".

Furthermore, these "families of similar compounds" can include literally hundreds of separate and similar compounds so understanding how they work is challenging

Bad News in 2012

As research on the Antioxidants and their health benefits gathered pace a test called the "Oxygen Radical Absorbance Capacity" or "ORAC Test" was developed by the US Department of Agriculture. This test provided a measure of a food's antioxidant effect. Suddenly specific foods like Blueberries became "super foods" because of their excellent antioxidant content.

But following further research, the test was withdrawn in 2012 because the antioxidant effect seen in the laboratory, the "in vitro" effect, was not replicated in the body.

This seemed like a body blow to the whole argument that eating more fresh vegetables and fruits provided a richer, more diverse nutritional food source with wide health benefits.

Great News in 2013 –

Thank goodness for Balz Frei, professor and director, and his team at the Linus Pauling Institute, **Oregon State University** (OSU). In research conducted in conjunction with the American Heart Association Foundation and the National Institutes of Health, they observed that the "in vitro" antioxidant properties of Flavonoids did indeed have little or no value in the human body.

This was reported in a summary press release by David Stauth, (2009) in which Balz Frei, Emeritus Professor at Oregon State University, **(Online Source 24**), states:

> *"However, these same compounds may indeed benefit human health, but for reasons that are quite different – the body sees them as foreign compounds, researchers say, and through different mechanisms, they could play a role in preventing cancer or heart disease.*
>
> *Based on this new view of how flavonoids work, a relatively modest intake of them – the amount you might find in a healthy diet with five to nine servings of fruits and vegetables – is sufficient. Large doses taken via dietary supplements might do no additional good; an apple a day may still be the best bet".*

So, the "ORAC Test" was re-instated in 2013, along with the whole argument that eating more fresh fruits, vegetables and salads provided a richer more diverse nutritional food source with wide health benefits.

The lesson then and now is that the science is only just starting to unravel how things work at the molecular level.

What is really exciting about this research is that it is happening right now. The team at Oregon State University, together with others around the world are gradually unlocking some of the science of both the food we eat and how our bodies respond.

An Apple a Day and the "5 a Day" Rule

There are two particularly interesting points from the report by Balz Frei, Emeritus Professor at Oregon State University, in which he suggests:

> A healthy diet includes "five to nine servings of fruits and vegetables."
>
> Research indicates that the body is well adapted to utilize the micronutrients in fresh produce, just taking what it needs.

Well nine servings a day probably seems like quite a challenge. But we can take David Stauth's suggestion that "an apple a day may still be the best bet" and start to fine tune this so that we start our daily nutrition with:

- 5 servings of non-starchy vegetables and fruits

Now of course, other Foods like grains, legumes and starchy vegetables can also contain significant levels of our Vital Nutrients. So, any portions of these in the daily nutrition will add servings 6-9.

This takes me back to my original goal with Dr Younis. After including my "5 a day" from non-starchy vegetables and fruits, then everything else was a bonus. And of course, the non-starchy vegetables and fruits require minimal preparation, so they retain so many other nutrients like essential vitamins and minerals. These foods also supply a portion of our daily Carb energy requirement as well. But even so, why "5 a Day"?

Does the Science Really Support the "5 a Day" Rule?

I have referred to the WHO guidelines and to the research from Oregon State University, but actually the scientific evidence supporting the "5 a Day" Rule is a bit thin.

In fact, as Jayne Buxton, in her fascinating Book *"The Great Plant-Based Con"* **(Ref 9),** has this to say on page 71:

> *"According to Dr Harcombe it had it's beginnings in California in 1991 as a public-service partnership between the National Cancer Institute (NCI) AND Produce for Better Health Foundation, the sponsors list for which included specialist fruit and vegetable companies, general produce farms and chemical companies producing seeds, fungicides and insecticides. Five-a day was, essentially a marketing campaign"*

It seems there may have been some anticipation that the rationale might be supported by research to show how such an approach could help reduce incidents of cancer. But as Jayne Buxton explains, the research failed to support this hypothesis.

Now I don't want to get tangled in the argument over the merits or otherwise of a diet based solely on "Plant-based" foods. But Jayne Buxton does go on to say:

> *Dr. Harcombe maintains that eating five portions of fruits and vegetables a day is only beneficial to health (and for addressing obesity) if the fruit and vegetables are eaten in place of processed junk rather than instead of meat, fish, dairy, eggs and other highly nutritious foods"*

So perhaps the concept that we eat certain foods to try to mitigate disease rather misses the point. And another way to look at this is to consider that the range of nutrients, be they Phytochemicals or specific Antioxidants found in fruits and vegetables, but **NOT** in highly processed foods provide a complexity that we are only just starting to understand. And this complexity offers health benefits.

This very point is suggested by T. Colin Campbell in his sweeping book, *"The China Study"*, **(Ref 10).** Indeed, he suggests 8 Principles of Food and Health, the first of which is:

> **"Principle #1 Nutrition represents the combined activities of countless food substances. The whole is greater than the sum of its parts."**

He elaborates as follows:

> *"The main message I am trying to get across is this: the chemicals we get from the foods we eat are engaged in a series of reactions that work in concert to produce good health. These chemicals are carefully orchestrated by intricate*

> *controls within our cells and all through our bodies, and these controls decide what nutrient goes where, how much of each nutrient is needed and when each reaction takes place".*

And this leads us back to Balz Frei's observations regarding five to nine servings of fruits and vegetables, but especially to:

> Research indicates that the body is well adapted to utilize the micronutrients in fresh produce, just taking what it needs.

So, while the scientific evidence for "5 a Day" might indeed **be thin**, the rule does still have much merit in the same way that the "ORAC Test" is still valid, just for different reasons.

Vital Nutrients and Why I Endorse the "5 a Day" Rule

The easiest way I can endorse the "5 a Day" Rule is as follows:

> I find that I agree with Balz Frei's suggestion of 5 – 9 servings daily because this encourages both variety and sufficient amounts of fruits and vegetables to provide a wide range of health promoting nutrients
>
> I find that I agree with Dr Harcombe that eating plenty of fruits and vegetables in preference to highly processed foods does seem very sensible
>
> I find that I agree with both T. Colin Campbel's Principle #1 and his rational the wide range of nutrients "work in concert to produce good health".

And I would go further and include the benefits offered by our fibres.

> Both soluble and insoluble fibres play vital roles enabling efficient digestion and absorption of the food we eat, and especially as the food passes through the Small Intestine
>
> Both Soluble and Insoluble Fibres also play vital roles as Prebiotics feeding our Microbiome and helping to maintain a healthy balance in the different Microbiota throughout the digestive tract

But the real clincher for me is:

> Research indicates that the body is well adapted to utilize the micronutrients in fresh produce, just taking what it needs.

And I make no apology for repeating this numerous times because this highlights how we should all strive to eat a diet that works with the body. And if we do that then the body will take what it needs.

So, I feel the argument to endorse the "5 a Day" Rule is rather like the argument to re-introduce the "ORAC Test".

Throughout this Section I have described a wide range of nutrients that I refer to as Vital Nutrients. These include Phytochemicals & Antioxidants, Soluble & Insoluble Fibres and Probiotics & Prebiotics.

We might not know exactly how and why they help support good health, but the empirical evidence indicates that they do. Furthermore, it seems that the diversity of all the vital nutrients plays a key role.

Much as the initial rational for the "ORAC Test" was found wanting, the benefits of Antioxidants were real, but they just worked in a different way. And exactly how they work is still to be determined.

We might not have a specific list of vital nutrients or understand how they interact, but what we do know is that including a wide range of the Vital Nutrients in our diet does seem to help promote good health.

It is still important to bear in mind that the suggestion to include 5 – 9 servings of fruits and vegetables isn't prescriptive as such, but does serve two purposes by providing:

1. A wide range of all the different nutrients
2. A way to experiment and find the actual amounts that work for you

Due to my own medical history, it seems that I need "very generous portions" of vegetables to achieve my optimum diet. But that's just me. We all need to experiment to find the portion sizes that work best for ourselves.

I would add the caveat that I find it better to include a bit more non-starchy veg and maybe a bit more fruit than I need rather than too little. They are satiating and help to reduce the amount of concentrated Carb Foods I might otherwise include. And I find the "5 a Day" Rule is a catchy and easy way to remind myself of this every day.

•

21 Have we lost our way?

As I reflected back on my darkest times when my small intestines were not working, I felt I had completely lost my way with my own nutrition. But surprisingly, as I became more aware of how my base nutrients worked, I began to see this as a much wider issue.

For example, back in Chapter 15 I highlighted how the USDA recommends a daily amount of both Fibres for adults up to the age of 50 as follows:

25 grams for women

38 grams for men

Yet on average American adults eat just 10-15 grams a day! I suspect this is the case here in the UK and I was guilty too. Even after discovering the benefits of including plenty of Soluble and Insoluble Fibres in my diet, I still let it slip again!

Then in Chapter 19 I introduced a couple of quotes from S Bengmark, **(Online Source 23),** remarking on the apparent health benefits of fermented foods that we humans have developed and eaten over thousands if not hundreds of thousands of years.

And yet many modern fermenting methods have somehow reduced the benefits of these foods to the point that many modern pickled foods no longer contain the probiotics of their predecessors.

It seems there are all sorts of reasons or situations arising from the Modern Farmer Diet that can cause us to lose our way.

In the next Part we explore the foods we actually eat, the Food Groups, and how these have evolved to create the Modern Farmer Diet. It may come as a surprise how we have lost our way through some unintended consequences.

Part 4 – The Foods we eat

22. The Foods we all eat – Food Groups

The foods we eat can be categorized into Food Groups based on their source and the content of Food Types. Most Food Groups are a combination of two or more of the macronutrients plus other Food Types in varying amounts. We will use the classifications listed below and shown again on **Table 9** shortly.

This list is subjective of course, but towards the top the foods have a higher protein content, in the middle they have higher levels of carbohydrates and towards the bottom they have higher levels of vital nutrients, as follows:

- **Meat, Fish & Eggs**
- Concentrated plant proteins, Tofu & Quorn
- Tree Nuts & Seeds
- Legumes & Pseudo-cereals, Soya Beans & Quinoa
- Grains like rice, wheat, spelt, maize and processed derivatives like bread and pasta
- Starchy Vegetables like potatoes, sweetcorn & yams
- Fruits
- Non-Starchy Vegetables, Salads (and Mushrooms)
- **Milk & Dairy**

Top and Bottom – A Classification for Everyone

This classification also caters for anyone following a vegan or vegetarian diet.

Foods from the Groups highlighted at the top and bottom can be included, or not. With attention to detail, the remaining Groups should be able to provide most of the base nutrients just about anyone needs. However, it is important to bear in mind that special care is required for some nutrients including Vitamins B12 & D and the Long Chain Fatty Acids DHA & EPA.

But the truth is, whatever our individual food preferences, we all need to take a little bit of care.

On **Table 9** over the page, we can see that Milk & Dairy is a mix of all three macronutrients. However, these foods are relatively new additions to the human diet and lactose intolerance is surprisingly widespread.

Whilst Milk & Dairy foods can make up a significant proportion of some diets around the world, especially the "Western" diet, they are completely absent in other diets.

Some Vegetarians may include "Milk & Dairy" Foods and even Eggs. But Vegans and stricter Vegetarians exclude these from their diet altogether.

Of course, the exact mix of nutrients varies between foods in each Group. So, **Table 9** is just intended to provide a "quick and easy visual estimate" of the nutrition content of the different Food Groups.

It is not perfect. Some sources refer to peas as vegetables, others refer to peanuts as nuts, but of course, they are both legumes. Then what about cashews? Where do they fit in?

There are a lot of grey areas when it comes to nutrition. The boundaries can be fluid and new research appears all the time.

And no matter how we try to categorize our food there will always be exceptions.

But this is half the fun! The lists in all the categories are deliberately short so you can get started adding your own.

Food Groups	Examples	Carb Energy	Fat Energy	Protein
Meat, Fish and Eggs	Beef, chicken, pork, lamb, game, cod, salmon, crab, eggs		●	⬤
Concentrated plant/fungus protein	Tofu (curdled soybeans). Tempeh (fermented soybean), Quorn	•	●	⬤
Tree Nuts and Seeds	Walnuts, Brazil, Cashew, Sesame, Sunflower, Flax,		⬤	●
Legumes and Pseudo-cereals	Lentils, Peas, beans, peanuts, chickpeas, quinoa, buckwheat, amaranth	⬤	●	•
Grains and derivatives	Wheat, spelt oats, rice, bread, pasta,	⬤	•	•
Starchy vegetables	Potatoes, yams, carrots, parsnips, sweet corn	⬤	○	○
Fruits	Apples, pears, plums, oranges, peaches, mango, berries, bananas	●	○	
Non-starchy vegetables salads, mushrooms	Cabbage, kale, broccoli, spinach cauliflower, peppers, lettuce, radish, onions, garlic mushrooms,	•		
Milk & Dairy	Milk, yoghurt, cheese, cottage cheese, butter	●	⬤	●

Table 9 A Quick & Fun Overview of the Food Groups and their main constituent Food Types

Vitamin	Mineral	Insoluble Fibres	Soluble Fibres	Antioxidant	Sensible portions provide a proportion of your daily requirement
•	•			●	
○	○	○	○	●	Significant ⬤
•	•	•	○	•	Healthy ●
•	•	•	•	•	Modest •
○	○	•	•	•	Low ○
•	•	•	•	•	
●	●	●	●	⬤	
●	●	⬤	⬤	⬤	
•	•			•	

Table 9 Continued

23. Exploring the Food Groups

Exploring the Food Groups

Now let's explore the Food Groups. To help us do this we can consider them in terms of four categories as shown in Table 10 on the following page.

Three categories are defined by their relative amounts of Proteins compared to their Energy content, from the Carbs and Fats. The fourth is defined by high levels of "Vital Nutrients", including soluble & insoluble fibres, antioxidants & phytochemicals, probiotics & prebiotics.

We start with the Food Groups in the High Protein category.

Category 1 - Meat, Fish and Eggs

By their very nature these are animal derived foods. It is significant that they contain relatively high levels of protein compared to most plant-based foods. As such we can treat them as **high protein foods**.

Many of these foods also provide "Complete Proteins". The impact of this combination becomes apparent when we start to count our proteins in Chapter 27.

In addition to the proteins, the different foods in this Group provide a variety of vitamins, minerals and other nutrients.

Of course, there are some nutritional downsides to any Food Group. So, with the Meat, Fish & Egg Group some products can be high in saturated fats and poorly farmed products may contain high levels of chemicals such as antibiotics or growth stimulants.

But if you do eat foods from this Group, you might be surprised to find that the quantities you need to meet your genuine daily protein requirements are modest. The body will utilize the amino acids in our diet very efficiently, if you let it.

Category	Description	Origin	Food Groups
1. High Protein	These are foods with the highest levels of Protein	Animal	-Meat, Fish & Egg
		Plant	-Concentrated Plant Protein
2. Protein +Energy	Foods with relatively high Protein but similar or higher levels of energy, often derived from Fats or Oils as well as Carbs.	Animal	-Milk & Dairy
		Plant	-Tree Nuts & Seeds -Legumes & Pseudo-cereals
3. High Energy + some Protein	Foods with high Energy levels, typically from Starchy Carbs. They may contain modest to low levels of Proteins.	Plant	-Grains & Derivatives -Starchy Vegetables
4. High Vitals +some Energy	Foods with high levels of different Vital Nutrients and energy mainly as simple Carbs	Plant	-Fruits -Non-Starchy Vegetables & Salads

Table 10. Four Categories of the Food Groups

(I refer to Category 3 as my Concentrated Carb Foods)

So maybe there is a place for small-scale, ethically managed livestock farming in our modern world. And if you choose not to eat animal products or dairy products, then there are many sources to find out how to achieve your own balanced diet with plant-based foods which we will come to shortly.

Category 1 - Concentrated Plant and Fungus Proteins

Although many plant-based foods do contain some protein, the levels are generally lower than the "Meat, Fish & Egg" Group. Furthermore, only a small number of single item plant-based foods provide "Complete Proteins".

I should add that different combinations of single plant foods can be combined to provide "Complete Proteins", but we will come back to these points in due course.

For the moment, we are comparing the options for plant-based, processed foods made from a single plant source that provide Complete Proteins with a total level of protein comparable with foods from the "Meat, Fish and Eggs" Group. With the increasing popularity of vegetarian and vegan diets more new food products may emerge, but currently there are only three widely available options, as follows:

> **Tofu –** Many people will be familiar with Tofu which originated in China and became a staple food across much of Asia. It was available in London by the 1770's and in the USA by the 1870's.
>
> It is derived from Soybeans, or Soya Beans whichever you prefer, and is prepared in a similar process to cheese making. Soy milk is coagulated to produce a curd like product. This is then pressed into solid white blocks.
>
> The process can be adapted to produce varying levels of softness from soft right up to extra firm. The end-product even looks like a soft but firm cheese.
>
> **Tempeh** – This is a less well-known soy product originating in Indonesia. Tempeh is produced by fermenting the Soybeans. This is then compacted into a firm cake like end product. Whilst Tofu has little flavour Tempeh has a distinct nutty

flavour and you can find out more in Kaitlyn Berkheiser's article titled "What's the difference between Tempeh and Tofu?" published online **(Online Source 25).**

Quorn - A new product, **Quorn** was developed and launched here in the UK as recently as 1985. It is derived from a specific type of fungus, or rather the soil mould Fusarium venenatum strain PTA-2684, first identified in a soil sample from a field by the River Thames near the town of Marlow in the UK.

The Fusarium venenatum strain PTA-2684 is grown in large fermentation vats with continuously oxygenated water to produce a Mycoprotein. The end-product is a little like soft Tofu or soft cheese in consistency.

Tofu, Tempeh and Quorn all contain "Complete Proteins" and can be used instead of "Meat or Fish" in all sorts of dishes.

Category 2 - Tree Nuts & Seeds

Whilst Tree Nuts and Seeds are not generally eaten in large enough quantities to be regarded as staple foods, they are still an important Food Group.

They contain relatively high levels of protein, although they are rarely complete proteins. But this means they are a great way to add diversity to protein in-take for everyone.

The different nuts and seeds across the whole Group provide a range of Vitamins, Minerals and Fibres. Furthermore, like Grains they can be harvested and stored with relative ease.

As a Group, they have a relatively high fat content. This includes a combination of what are generally regarded as healthier fats like monounsaturated and polyunsaturated fats together with low levels of saturated fats.

The saturated fats include Medium Chain Triglycerides or MCTs, which have a shorter triglyceride chain compared to most animal fats. There is some indication that the MCTs may be healthier, but as yet there is no definitive scientific proof. We'll come back to this in Chapter 28.

The combination of fats found in seeds like rapeseed (also called canola), hemp, cottonseed and sunflower make them a great and versatile source of vegetable oils. These oils are often used as a replacement for traditional cooking fats including dairy products like butter or meat products like dripping or lard which often have high levels of saturated fats.

But the Group, and particularly the seeds used for vegetable oil production, presents us with a dilemma. The ratio of the two parent polyunsaturated fats, Omega 3 and Omega 6 in the human diet should be somewhere between 1:1 and 1:4. However, the nuts and especially the seeds can have much higher levels of Omega 6.

So, whilst the good fats may offer health benefits like helping to lower harmful levels of LDL Cholesterol, there is emerging evidence that a sharp rise in the level of Omega 6 in the diet may disrupt the optimal ratio between Omega 3 and Omega 6.

This is just something to bear in mind and Kris Gunnars presents an interesting overview in her article titled "How to Optimize Your Omega-6 and Omega-3 Ratio" published online with Healthline: **(Online Source 26).**

Category 2 - Legumes & Pseudo-cereals

As a Group, these foods contain a high level of Carbohydrate and much of this is starchy carbohydrate. They can also contain a combination of monounsaturated and polyunsaturated fats together with low levels of saturated fats. But the total fat content is generally lower than for the "Tree Nuts & Seeds" Group.

These are high energy foods and many also contain a relatively high protein content for plant-based foods. These are great foods for anyone following a Vegetarian or Vegan diet.

The list goes on because many of these foods also contain a range of vitamins and minerals as well as high levels of fibres. And for more information check out the article by Lizzie Streit and Ruairi Robertson titled "9 Healthy Beans and Legumes You Should Try", **(Online Source 27).**

The range of different foods in this Group is considerable and the diversity of cooking options they offer is just wonderful. They are a great addition to everyone's diet.

> **Legumes** include all sorts of beans like kidney, soya and black beans, chickpeas, peas, lentils and peanuts. The last is often mistakenly referred to as a nut and likewise, peas are often mistakenly referred to as vegetables. The dried seed of the legumes are also called Pulses and some legumes can even be considered a type of fruit.
>
> With the notable exception of Soya Beans, peas and peanuts, the Legumes do not provide "Complete Proteins". But different legumes and other plant proteins can be mixed, and the combinations can provide "Complete Proteins", as we cover again in Chapter 27.
>
> **Pseudo-Cereals** are so called because even though the foods are seeds rather than grains, they can be used in much the same way as cereals. They are particularly important for Vegetarians and Vegans because some of these can contain "Complete Proteins",
>
> The three well known varieties are Quinoa, Buckwheat and Amaranth. Both Buckwheat and Amaranth can be used to make types of bread

Like the Grains, many foods in this group can be harvested, transported and stored with minimal processing.

Relatively modest amounts can provide most of your daily energy requirements and a significant amount of protein as well.

They are an important Group in the **Modern Farmer Diet** and like the grains they have played a major role in the development of civilizations around the world.

Category 3 - Grains

The Grains contain high levels of Carbohydrate and much of this is starchy carbohydrate. These are energy foods and if there is one Food Group that symbolizes the **"Modern Farmer Diet"** this is it.

It is the capacity of the grains to be cultivated, harvested, stored and transported with minimal processing that makes them the signature Food Group of the **Modern Farmer Diet**. Of course, there are other comparable foods, but Grains somehow encapsulate the whole progression from Hunter Gatherer Societies to Modern Civilizations based on Farmed Foods. Let's start by considering them in terms of preparation:

> **Simple Preparation** - There are grains like rice, oats, corn and maize that we can eat in simple cooked forms.
>
> **More Involved Preparation** - And there are grains like wheat, spelt and barley that are more often used in derivatives like bread and pasta. And of course, corn can be used to make tortillas.

There are numerous other grains grown around the world, but the different types and varieties of grain are too numerous to cover here. Their role in the development of civilizations and the population of the world is best symbolized by Rice and Wheat:

> **Rice -** This amazing grain is the staple food for more than half of the world's population. According to Ricepedia.org "Rice provided 19% of global human per capita energy and 13 % of per capita protein in 2009".
>
> **Wheat –** This grain provides the staple food for a more modest 35% of the world's population. But according to the International Development Research Centre, IDRC, wheat "provides more calories and protein in the world's diet than any other crop".

There is an interesting overview on the IDRC website titled "Facts & Figures on Food and Biodiversity, **(Online Source 28).** The contribution of these two grains is quite remarkable.

It is also easy to think of the grains just in terms of human consumption, but a significant percentage of the world's grain production is now used for livestock feed. In Europe and North America crops like Barley, Rye and Oats are particularly important.

Across Asia a significant percentage of the Maize crop is used for livestock feed as is the Sorghum crop in parts of Africa.

It is fascinating to see how eating habits change. In the not-too-distant past Barley was originally grown for human consumption but it is now grown mainly for livestock feed. And crops like Maize and Sorghum are now being planted more widely in temperate climates for both livestock feed and human consumption.

As an aside though, it is interesting to note that older varieties like spelt seem to have higher protein contents. It seems that progress sometimes takes us down unintended paths.

Reflecting on my own diet, there are probably only occasional days when I don't include one or more grain products in my diet. Whenever possible I choose the whole grain products because these also provide a range of other nutrients including Vitamins, Minerals, Fibres, as well as small amounts of Protein.

But the foods in this Food Group pack a lot of energy. So first and foremost, I treat them as an important and prime source of energy. Then I consider the extra nutrients as a bonus.

Category 3 - Starchy Vegetables

The Starchy Vegetables are classified as such because they contain high levels of starchy carbohydrates.

Like the other High Energy Foods, including "Grains", "Legumes and Pseudo-Cereals", the "Starchy Vegetables" need to be cooked to make that energy available. Indeed, many are completely inedible in the raw state. But the preparation and cooking process is generally quite simple.

However, their capacity to be stored for any length of time is considerably shorter than for "Grains" or "Legumes & Pseudo-Cereals" because they retain much of their moisture content. This also means they require more careful transportation and storage to avoid damaging the crop.

The High Energy content of the "Starchy Vegetables" means they are often important staple foods.

They also typically contain high levels of fibres together with various vitamins and minerals. But they have relatively low protein contents more typical of plant-based foods. They are, however, very versatile and lend themselves to all types of preparation and cooking.

The range of crops in this Food Group is quite modest and is dominated by the following:

Potatoes, sweet potatoes, sweetcorn, parsnips, yams, and winter squashes like pumpkins

The dominant crops in any region will be largely determined by suitability of growing conditions. So, Yams might be dominant in warmer climates and potatoes in cooler ones.

Just like the "Grains", the "Starchy Vegetables" are packed with energy, and I treat them primarily as an important source of energy. And I treat the other nutrients including Vitamins, Minerals, Fibres and Proteins as a bonus.

Category 4 - Non-Starchy Vegetables and Fruits

I have lumped the non-Starchy Vegetables and Fruits together because it is actually quite difficult to separate them out.

Any keen gardener will be aware you can categorize vegetables and fruits in terms of their plant family. These include cabbage, squash, legume and so on using the common names rather than full Latin nomenclature. But even these can be confusing.

The classification of fruits is certainly fun. For example, Blueberries are Berries, but Strawberries are not. On the other hand, Peaches, Coconuts and Olives are not three fruits you might lump together and yet they are all Drupes.

However, another approach is to categorize them on the basis of the part of the plant we eat. This approach is helpful because it also highlights the different nutritional value of all sorts of plant foods.

Table 11a on the following page lists the parts of the plant where the different vegetables and fruits are found. The Table also presents a "rough & ready" visual estimate of the nutrient content.

It is subjective of course and there are lots of "anomalies". For example, the category "Roots and Tubers" illustrates a key issue. Some of the plants here like Potatoes and Sweet Potatoes are in the "Starchy Vegetable" Food Group but others like Carrots and Parsnips are closer to the non-Starchy classification with much lower energy content.

The list of examples just scratches the surface because there are so many more vegetables and fruits. There are also many varieties of each as well. But it does illustrate just how many nutrients the foods in this Category provide. They are the star foods in our diet.

And to complicate things, some of these may even be described as "Salads" because they can be used raw in cold food preparations.

We can be overwhelmed by this selection and choice, or we can find ways to explore and experiment. You can use this initial list to get you started. And you can use the visual estimate of nutritional value to help you along the way.

Finally, before we leave this Category/Group, I want to flag up an issue or rather a question that seems to pop up quite regularly:

Does fruit make you fat?

Well actually there is something in this. We raise it again in the following Chapter and address it in detail in Chapter 30.

Category 2 - Milk & Dairy

Foods from the "Milk & Dairy" Group may be common in some geographic regions and cultures and totally absent in others.

Cattle are the most commonly used animal for milk and dairy production. But other animals include Water Buffalo, Goat, Sheep, Camel, Donkey, Horse, Reindeer and Yak.

Plant Part	Examples	Energy	Vits& Mins	Fibres	Anti-Oxidants
Fruits	Sub acid - apple, stone fruit, oranges	●	⬤	●	⬤
	Berry and Berry like –, Blueberries, Grapes strawberry, Cranberry,	●	⬤	●	⬤
	Starchy, alkali and fatty like avocado, olive, banana, dates	●	●	●	●
	Savoury Fruit like tomato, bell peppers, pumpkin, cucumber	•	●	●	⬤
Flowers and Buds	Broccoli, Green Beans, Cauliflower, Courgettes, Sweet Peas	○	●	●	⬤
Leaves	Cabbage, Kale, Spinach, Water Cress, Lettuce, Chard	○	•	⬤	⬤
Stalks and Stems	Celery, Asparagus, Rhubarb, Kohlrabi, Leek	○	●	⬤	●
Bulbs	Onions, Shallots, Garlic,	○	●	⬤	⬤
Roots and Tubers	Potatoes, Beets, Carrots, Turnips, Sweet Potatoes, Yams, Parsnip**	⬤	●	●	●
Fungi	Mushrooms, truffles,	○	•	○	○

Table 11a A Quick & Fun Overview of the Non-Starchy Vegetables and Fruits

***Potatoes, Sweet Potatoes and Yams are Starchy Vegetables of course, but some other Roots & Tubers are Non-Starchy Vegetables.*

Sensible portions provide this proportion of your daily requirement	Significant	Healthy	Modest	Low
	⬤	●	•	○

Table 11b A Visual Scale for 11a

Quite how humans came to treat the milk of other animals as a food source is lost in the mists of time. But the end result is a wide selection of different foods including:

Milk, Yoghurt, Cheese, Butter, Whey

These in turn may be used to produce more food that may be referred to as Dairy Products.

In terms of nutrients, milk and many dairy products can contain a fairly even amount of all three macronutrients, carbs, fats and proteins. The latter are generally "Complete Proteins". The precise ratio can be adjusted or manipulated by different processes to produce foods like Whey Proteins, Low fat milk or Casein rich Cottage Cheese.

Milk and dairy products can also be a good source of calcium, potassium and magnesium as well as Vitamins A, B2, B12 and D.

And with the growing interest in regenerative farming and Grass Fed Beef, it is interesting to note that milk from Grass Fed cows and butter made from such milk can also contain modest amounts of DHA and EPA, the important Long Chain Omega 3 Fatty Acids. We will revisit this issue again in Chapter 31, page 210.

However, one specific dietary drawback to these foods is an intolerance to lactose, a specific sugar found in most animal milk and particularly cow's milk.

Depending on your own food preferences I shall leave it to you to decide if you want to include these in your diet or not.

Food Groups and Covering your Food Types

With such a range of food choices how do we start to pick out the best food choices to satisfy our own individual needs?

Our personal food choices may be guided by:

- Age and Gender
- Our level of physical activity
- Food preferences, including omnivore, carnivore, pescatarian, vegetarian and vegan choices.
- Religious beliefs
- Affordability
- Access to different foods
- Intolerances and allergies
- Even medical conditions

No matter what guidelines shape our personal choices, we all need to cover all our base nutrients, in other words all our Food Types.

As I suggested earlier, we can use the Four Key Categories of Food Groups to help us pick our way through this vast range of food choices, so Table 10 is shown again on the opposite page for quick reference.

Ever-Expanding Food Choices

But we need to take a step back for a moment. It appears that the Modern Farmer Diet has expanded the food options for many of us with a vast range of food choices across all the Food Groups. This could be a source of confusion because:

> **The base nutrients or Food Types we all need in our diet haven't changed over time. But the foods we eat, our Food Groups, have changed significantly.**

Category	Description	Origin	Food Groups
1. High Protein	These are foods with the highest levels of Protein	Animal	- Meat, Fish & Egg
		Plant	- Concentrated Plant Protein
2. Protein +Energy	Foods with relatively high Protein but similar or higher levels of energy, often derived from Fats or Oils as well as Carbs.	Animal	-Milk & Dairy
		Plant	-Tree Nuts & Seeds -Legumes & Pseudo-cereals
3. High Energy + some Protein	Foods with high Energy levels, typically from Starchy Carbs. They may contain modest to low levels of Proteins.	Plant	-Grains & Derivatives -Starchy Vegetables
4. High Vitals +some Energy	Foods with high levels of different Vital Nutrients and energy mainly as simple Carbs	Plant	-Fruits -Non-Starchy Vegetables & Salads

Table 10 (Again). Four Categories of the Food Groups

(I refer to Category 3 as my Concentrated Carb Foods)

And change continues at a pace. Modern farming and food production methods combined with transport, processing and storage all continue to evolve providing us with an ever-growing range of foods from which to choose.

Furthermore, with such a wide range of foods now available to us, maybe we have forgotten how to pick our way through the huge choice. And as the range of foods continues to expand, it is getting even more difficult to achieve our own optimum diet.

I have included Table 10 again because it provides a simple overview of the Food Groups and how they fit into the 4 categories. You might find this handy when you start afresh planning your meals.

This is a good moment to pause to consider how the Modern Farmer Diet evolved and look at some of the unintended consequences of this process.

24. Evolution and the Modern Farmer Diet

The Modern Farmer Diet

The vast range of foods across the Food Groups reflects the development of what we can call the **Modern Farmer Diet**.

There are some societies still following a Hunter Gatherer lifestyle and diet, but these are the exceptions in the modern world. So, I am using the name as a generalized term for all the diets around the world largely based on farming and agriculture.

The **Modern Farmer Diet** can take many forms because people from different regions, climates and cultures have developed different livestock and a vast range of crops that can be cultivated and processed to create nutritious foods.

Perhaps this all started when our early ancestors found basic cooking and processes like drying and smoking enhanced the level of nutrition they obtained from meats and fish as well as increasing the length of time the processed foods could be stored for.

Or maybe it started as cooking and other basic processes were used to convert previously inedible plants like root tubers and seeds into very nutritious foods. Or perhaps they happened side by side. This is a fascinating area of research we will expand on shortly.

And as we reflect on the role of cooking and processed foods in the story of human evolution, it may be surprising to observe how some of the new food additions have ended up leading us to a strange place.

I personally feel that studying the evolution from the Hunter Gatherer Diet to the Modern Farmer Diet may help us make the most of our new-found abundance of choice and help us identify foods we should really treat with a little bit of care.

The rapid evolution of the Modern Farmer Diet

In his wonderful book *"Catching Fire – How cooking made us human"* **(Ref 11)**, leading anthropologist Professor Richard Wrangham, proposes the radical idea that our distant ancestors, Homo Erectus, started to cook meat and certain plants such as roots and tubers as far back 1.9-1.8 million years ago.

Professors Stephen Cunnane and Michael Crawford and others propose the idea that some 300-200,000 years ago the Homo Sapiens started to include cooked fish and seafood, **(Online Source 29)**. These foods are often a richer source of EPA and DHA than most meats. This boost in key Long Chain Fatty Acids may have contributed to the increased neural capacity of the modern human brain.

A further stage of processing in which barely edible foods like seeds are first ground, mixed with water and then baked to produce a type of food we now know as bread may have only begun some 40-30,000 years ago.

What we would recognize as organized agriculture emerged around 12,000 years ago. Then in a comparatively short period of time the new concepts of agriculture provide the ability to control our food supply. This fundamentally changes both our diet and the way we live. And this rapid evolution is summarized in Table 12 over three pages.

Of course, this is just the briefest summary following a few possible routes of evolution. Others suggest alternative routes of evolution and human development.

The introduction of new foods does demonstrate the ingenuity of humans all around the world. All sorts of leaves, seeds, fruits, tubers, stalks and bulbs have been adapted to produce nutritious foods. Quite how some processes came about really gives you pause for thought.

Take the familiar Olive as an example. The raw fruit is quite inedible because of the intensely bitter taste caused by the chemical compound called oleuropein.

How and why did our early ancestors work out that packing the olives in salt or soaking them in brine removed this chemical? However, it happened, and the result is a versatile food that has been widely cultivated for thousands of years.

1	**2.5 to 1.65 million years**	The **earliest Hominids,** including **Homo habilis,** were ape-like and lived in trees. They had a brain size of **approx. 1 lb.** As well as plants, fruit, and seeds there is evidence they cut animal meat from the bone. Are these the first true **"Hunter Gatherers?"**
2	**1.9/1.8 million years ago** ***Did they eat Cooked Meat, Roots, and Tubers? – our first processed foods***	**Homo Erectus** emerged as the first upright Hominids. With a larger cranial capacity and bigger brain, they were also taller and marked by a decrease in the size of the digestive system, mouth, and teeth. Do they represent the stage in evolution when our distant ancestors **started to cook meat, roots, and tubers,** as proposed by Prof Wrangham in his book Catching Fire? Cooked foods are digested more easily providing more nutrient value.
3	**800-600,000 years ago** ***Evidence of cooked Meat, Roots, and Tubers***	**Homo heidelbergensis** emerged. They were distinguished by a significantly bigger cranial capacity, the brain size increased to **approx. 3 lb.** The evidence grows that they too cooked food including meat, roots, and tubers.
4	**300-200,000 years ago** ***Compelling evidence of cooked Meat, Roots, and Tubers***	**Homo sapiens** emerged as our earliest direct ancestors. The brain size is comparable to our own, weighing **approx. 3 lbs**. The evidence is compelling that they ate a **"Hunter Gatherer Diet"** including cooked meat, roots, and tubers. A further line of research proposes that early Homo sapiens extended this diet to include fish and seafood both of which are rich in Omega 3 Long Chain Fatty Acids.

Table 12a Evolution of the Modern Farmer Diet

	...continued ***Introduction of Fish and Seafood which include Omega 3 Long Chain Fatty Acids***	Evidence points to 10-50% of the protein content of the diet being derived from seafood and fish. The hypothesis suggests these Omega 3s were critical to the development of the more complex brains that distinguish the Homo sapiens and are fundamental to being human today. Omega 3 Long Chain Fatty Acids, **EPA & DHA** make up about **8 % of the modern human brain.** Proposed by Prof Cunnane, this hypothesis is not widely accepted as yet. But it is an exciting area of research that may shed light on the importance of EPA and DHA in the modern diet.
5	**40-30,000 years ago (roughly)** ***Bread - A new supplement in times of need***	There is evidence of seeds and root tubers that were only partially edible when raw being pounded, ground, mixed with water and baked **to produce a type of bread.** This development in preparation and cooking appears to provide a new food to supplement the normal "Hunter Gatherer Diet" in times of need.
6	**12,000 years ago** ***Bread and other concentrated starchy carbohydrates become the new food staples***	Organized agriculture emerges in the Middle East from modern day Turkey to Egypt. This provides a regular source of grains like wheat, which is used to make bread and other types of concentrated starchy carbohydrate foods. These become the staple foods of new farmer societies. The new type of society and the **"Modern Farmer Diet"** start to displace hunter gatherer societies all around the world. But there is evidence of the rise of illness and disease in the new farmer societies.

Table 12b Evolution of the Modern Farmer Diet

7	**A - Less than 10,000 years ago** ***New processed foods have been added to the human diet.***	More cultivated grains and processed foods emerge in different cultures around the world including: 8,700 yrs. – Maize in Central America 8,000 yrs. – Rice in Asia and Africa 7,000 yrs. - Dairy foods in Europe 6,500 yrs. – Olive Oil in Eastern Med 2,500 yrs. – Sugar in India. Whilst some of these new processed foods expand the diet in a positive way, some others such as sugar are just for flavour and offer little nutritional value.
7	**B - Less than 150 years ago** ***More new processed foods are added at a fast rate.***	More processed foods are added including: 1. 1886 Kellogg's launch "Breakfast Cereals" 2. 1901 Hydrogenated oils or Trans Fats replace fats from animal sources. 3. 1916 Mastin's Yeast Vitamon Tablet's, possibly the first multi-vitamin product. 4. 1920s Packaged fresh orange juice from Florida. 5. 1960s High Fructose Corn Syrup developed as an alternative to sugar. 6. 1970s New concentrated oils from Rapeseed (or Canola) and later safflower and sunflower seeds. 7. 1985 - Quorn a new type of protein is developed by fermenting soil mould

Table 12c Evolution of the Modern Farmer Diet

We should also bear in mind that many of the large succulent fruits as well as many salads and vegetables grown so widely today are actually the result of relatively modern farming methods.

Indeed, many of the cultivation techniques used in modern agriculture are described in the works of Mago of Carthage some 4,500 years ago from the 3rd or 2nd century BC. So much so that Mago is often described as the Father of Agriculture. **(Online Source 30).**

So, it seems that much of our perception of large succulent fruits and vegetables may reflect foods that are actually quite a recent addition to our diet. We come back to this in Chapter 30.

Regardless of the exact line of evolution and change, the evidence, particularly over the last 12,000 years, does illustrates another key point:

> **We find that many staple foods of the "Modern Farmer Diet" including grains such as wheat, barley, maize and rice, derivatives like bread, pasta and tortillas and even many large succulent fruits are in fact, very recent additions to our diet.**

This evolutionary process in the cultivation and production of food has brought enormous benefits that have allowed civilizations to flourish. But at the same time, there may be a recurring theme that the new-found food stability has also brought with it society-wide health problems.

It seems that the Modern Farmer Diet can leave us in a strange place where we don't know how to take full advantage of our new choices. Perhaps some of the new foods added to the human diet have resulted in unintended consequences and we will explore some of these in the following Chapter.

25. The Modern Farmer Diet and unintended consequences

In a short period of time many new foods have been added to the human diet. Have they resulted in some unintended consequences?

Perhaps the most obvious of these unintended consequences in this modern day and age is the rise in obesity in many Western nations. Rising levels of obesity seem to go hand in hand with increased health issues such as diabetes, high blood pressure and heart disease.

Examining some of the new foods in terms of the **Food Groups** and the constituent **Food Types** may explain why their introduction may have had unintended consequences such as:

1. **Eating an energy dense and micronutrient poor diet** – this was recognized in the mid-1900s when synthetic vitamins were developed to supplement poor diets when fresh produce was out of season. And the situation persists through to the modern day. In the UK, for example, it is estimated that some 20-30% of the population are deficient in Vitamin D.

2. **Eating an excessively energy dense diet** – this may be one of the fundamental causes of the rising problem with obesity in this modern age and all the health problems that obesity and excess weight can trigger.

3. **Eating a diet lacking in both soluble and insoluble fibres** – despite advice from respected bodies such as the University of California, San Francisco, a significant percentage of the adult US population eat considerably less than the recommended daily intake of fibres. And I suspect the same is true for the UK as well.

4. **Pushing for Low Fat or No Fat diets** – yet the Omega 3s and Omega 6s are integral to being human with the Omega 3 Long Chain Fatty Acids making up some 8% of the dry weight of the brain. Furthermore, four of our essential vitamins are fat soluble, and fats should be an important source of energy too.

5. **Rising levels of food intolerances and allergies** – there is a growing awareness of food intolerance to some of the recent additions like gluten in wheat or lactose in milk. But the levels of intolerances and allergies may also be rising with foods like peanuts, tree nuts, shellfish and some fruits joining what seems like an ever-growing list.

6. **Introduction of new concentrated foods** – The new man-made Trans Fats have a different molecular structure to natural fats and may affect us at a cellular level. Could these man-made Trans Fats pose health issues that are yet to be fully recognized? And new seed oils such as rapeseed (canola) or sunflower oils contain much higher levels of Omega 6 relative to their Omega 3 content. Could we be creating yet another health issue?

7. **Racing to add completely new foods** – as the world population continues to grow there is enormous pressure to find new food sources. This may be particularly true for foods with a high protein content because these are lacking in so many diets worldwide. New sources have been introduced including insects and mycoproteins like Quorn. The latter was developed by fermenting a soil fungus found growing in a field by the River Thames. I'll leave you to decide if these options represent real progress or not.

This list is subjective of course and only highlights a few potential issues with the Modern Farmer Diet.

There does seem to be a recurring theme, that despite an expanding choice of foods, the Modern Farmer Diet has the potential to lead to a monotonous diet lacking key nutrients and especially micronutrients.

Perhaps we can generalize by suggesting that the changes allowed civilizations to flourish but gave us a "Modern Farmer Diet" that can sometimes be:

Energy rich and Micronutrient poor

Of course, this is not true of every modern diet around the world. These issues are not universal, nor are they necessarily fixed in time.

Some countries and societies, or groups, families or individuals within a country seem to enjoy high levels of vibrant good health on their Modern Farmer Diet and yet other countries or groups seem to flounder to some degree. These issues do, however, highlight two big questions:

- How can we **ALL** take advantage of the wonderful selection of modern foods?
- Which foods in our modern diet need to be treated with a little care?

It seems that our growing range of food choices comes with a bit of a catch.

Exploring our Macronutrients and Tackling the Calorie Conundrum

Before we can start looking at how to tackle the issue of a diet that is Micronutrient poor, we first need to explore our Macronutrients in more depth. And we need to understand why counting our calories might not be quite as straight forward as it may first appear. I will refer to this as:

The Calorie Conundrum

We explore our Macronutrients and the Calorie Conundrum in Part 5.

Part 5 – The Calorie Conundrum and our Macronutrients

26. Our Macronutrients and the Calorie Conundrum

What are Calories?

The term calorie is widely used as a measure of the energy content of food. Now that sounds simple enough, but as with everything to do with nutrition, there is some ambiguity. For a start there are two calories, the "**small calorie**" and the "**Large Calorie**".

The "small calorie" is the heat energy required to heat 1 gram of water by 1 degree Celsius. The "Large Calorie" is the heat energy required to raise the temperature of 1 kilogram of water by 1 degree Celsius. By convention, the food sciences and food industry use the "Large Calorie". However, in Food Labelling the "Large Calorie" may be referred to as:

Large Calorie or Cal
Food Calorie or calorie
Kilocalorie or kcal or even Kcal

To simplify things all references to calories or Calories in this book are to the "Large Calories". Now putting that to one side, the daily calorie count, or total energy content of the food we eat, is a useful tool. Indeed, the starting point for many "diets" is your daily calorie count. But counting our calories presents us with a conundrum.

Using Calorie Count to compare populations

The UK government guidelines for the daily calorie count, shown back in Chapter 8, are as follows:

- 2500 calories for the average adult male
- 2000 calories for the average adult female

The equivalent USDA guidelines recommend 2700 and 2200 calories respectively. And both sets of recommendations are averages for adults just going about their daily lives and individual recommendations will vary from one individual to another.

So, anyone engaged in a particularly active lifestyle will probably need more calories. Conversely, anyone leading a more sedate lifestyle will probably need less.

It seems that the calorie count is useful as a simple measure of energy to compare groups and populations. For example, the Food and Agricultural Organization (FAO) and the United Nations (UN) publish average calorie consumption across whole adult populations. UN Published results for 2022 are surprising, **(Online Source 31):**

- Average calories per person globally 2,960 per day
- Average calories per person across Europe and North America 3,540 per day

We can take data for the average calorie consumption across the whole adult populations of countries or regions and consider a question like:

Why is our average energy intake so high?

The data suggest either that the populations as a whole are very active, or that a lot of people are eating too much energy!

I am inclined to think it is probably the latter. Why? Well, if we review the Food Groups in Table 10 back on page 97, we see that the "Modern Farmer Diet" contains a lot of different high energy foods.

So, for those of us in the UK or the USA, the average energy intake figures indicate that we may need to take care with these foods so that we don't constantly exceed our genuine energy requirements.

Calories and all our Macronutrients

Now we need to work out how we can use the calorie count on an individual level. And I appreciate that there are different "apps" available, but it is useful to understand some of the underlying issues.

You will recall, from Page 38, that the daily calorie count may also be defined in terms of the ratio of macronutrients. Here in the UK the widely accepted recommendation is:

Recommended Daily Consumption as a % of Total Calories	Macronutrients		
	Carbs	Fats	Proteins
	50%	35%	15%

Table 13 Recommended Daily Macronutrient consumption

I haven't found the original source of this recommendation, but I was surprised to find it was used by the Commandos in the 1940s, as reported in *"The Commando Pocket Manual, 1940-1945"* I referred to earlier, **(Ref 3).**

I would also add that this fascinating manual has been reprinted and is available through regular book sources.

Back in the 1940s the original Commandos were a fit and healthy lot, just as their modern-day counterparts, the Royal Marines Commandos, are today. So, it is worth listening to what they have to say about nutrition.

The same Manual goes on to refer to Fats and Carbs as "fuel foods" and Proteins as "building materials".

The recommendation is that your daily proteins should make up some 15% of your daily calorie requirements. However, these calories are primarily used to build and maintain your skeletal muscle mass and are not used for energy as such.

And this raises and interesting question:

> **Does the ratio of macronutrients stay the same for different levels or types of activity?**

Apparently not, as Point 59 on Page 81 of the manual states:

> *59. Increased physical work demands an increase in the fuel foods, but not in the protein part of the ration.*

But that's not quite the whole story.

I discussed this issue with Toby Garbett who competed with the GB Rowing Team for 9 years, winning two world titles and competing at two Olympic Games, **(Ref A).** He pointed out that the athletes in training were eating between 5,000 and 6,000 Calories a day, day in and day out. And sometimes more.

Even if we use the lower figure of 5,000 Calories and the percentages in Table 13, 15% of 5,000 Calories would equate to 750 Calories. As Proteins provide 4 Calories per Gram, see Table 14, this equates to:

187.5 Grams of Protein per day

However, the level of Protein recommended to athletes was increased but it was not measured as the percentage of the increased total calorie count shown above.

Instead of using the 15% figure, the recommended protein count was measured by weight up to a maximum of 0.68 g per lb of Bodyweight (or 1.5 g per kg of Bodyweight) for both Male and Female athletes.

Now, as I will demonstrate in due course, the approach recommended to the athletes who are engaged in intense high-level training results in what can only be described as a modest increase in the amount of protein in the diet. But this was calculated as sufficient to maintain all the protein functions in the body as well as maintaining the skeletal muscle mass. Furthermore:

The increase in daily protein is less than maintaining the protein content as a set percentage of the total calorie count.

It seems that Point 59 from the Commando Manual is partly correct in that we should measure our proteins separately from our total calorie count. And the recommendation to the rowing athletes to use an amount of protein determined by bodyweight and activity level gives us a tool to do this.

So, our daily calorie count is more than just a simple measure of how much energy we need. The calorie count includes both the building materials we need, our proteins, and the energy we need, our Carbs and Fats. It seems that the ratio of these three nutrients can vary depending on the level and type of activity we are engaged in.

This is a really important point which we will cover in more detail shortly, but before we do there is another issue.

Calculating the Calorie Count for our Food Intake

Putting aside the issue of the ratio of macronutrients for a moment, we also find that just trying to measure all our macronutrients to calculate our daily calories can be quite a challenge. Again, I appreciate there are "apps" available, but it is still useful to explore the detail.

For a start, when we are preparing food, we don't usually measure it out by the calorie content of the macronutrients. We usually measure it by weight and sometimes by volume. Most of the time it is by weight, so we need to know the approximate calorific value of each of macronutrients by weight, as follows:

Calorific Value of the Macros as:	Macronutrient		
	Carbs	Fats	Proteins
Calories per Gram	4	9	4

Table 14 Calorific Value of the Macronutrients

That all sounds easy enough! But we must also take account of the different measuring systems, Pounds and Ounces or Kilograms and Grams.

And let's not forget measures like Tablespoons and Teaspoons. A lot of sources like diet books or recipe books happily switch between the different measuring systems which can be confusing.

Anyway, once we know the weight of each macronutrient in any food portion we are eating, we can work out the number of calories of each of our macronutrients and then the daily total calorie count.

And then we can work out the percentages. Right? **PHEW!!**

The calorie count seems deceptively simple and yet it is far more involved and nuanced than just a simple measure of energy. And calculating your count on a daily basis is quite an involved process.

Using the Calorie Count on a Day-to-Day Basis

So, what happens when we try to use the calorie count and ratio of macronutrients on a day-to-day basis?

The guideline calorie count and ratio of macronutrients introduced above are fine **IF** we are roughly average weight and our day-to-day activity level is more or less in line with some notional population average. And that it stays around that level day in and day out.

But what if we are heavier or lighter than the national average. And what if our activity level:

- Is significantly higher or lower than this notional average.
- Fluctuates significantly from day to day.

We can explore the effect by using estimates of my daily calorie requirements across a typical week. These estimates are shown in Table 15 below.

Day	Activity	Activity Level	Daily Calories
Monday	Work + Strength w/o	Physically Active	3,100
Tuesday	Work + General Stuff	Average	2,500
Wednesday	Work + Strength w/o	Physically Active	3,100
Thursday	Work + General Stuff	Average	2,500
Friday	Work + Strength w/o	Physically Active	3,100
Saturday	Big Run + Family Stuff	Physically Active	3,200
Sunday	Recovery Run + Fam Stuff	Physically Active	3,100
Daily Average over the Week			**2,9430**

Table 15 Estimated Activity Levels and Daily Calories

And as you can see, my calorie requirements vary quite significantly from one day to the next. But rather than just estimating my protein requirement as 15% of my total calories I set out to take into account both my bodyweight and the varying levels of activity for each day.

Now I do need to jump ahead here and introduce Table 16 below.

Protein Requirement for Female aged 40			
Bodyweight in lbs ***in kgs***	**1** USDA Min requirement 0.33 g/lb 0.72 g/kg	**2** Physically active requirement 0.51 g/lb 1.12 g/kg	**3** Top level sport requirement 0.68 g/lb 1.5 g/kg
100lbs ***45.5kg***	**33 g**	**50.5 g**	**68 g**
<u>120lbs</u> ***54.5kg***	**<u>39.6 g</u>**	**<u>60.6 g</u>**	**81.6 g**
140lbs ***63.6kg***	**46.2 g**	**70.7 g**	**95.2 g**
160lbs ***72.7kg***	**52.8 g**	**80.8 g**	**108.8 g**
180lbs ***81.8kg***	**59.4 g**	**90.9 g**	**122.4 g**
200lbs ***90.6kg***	**66 g**	**101 g**	**136 g**
Protein Requirement for Male aged 40			
Bodyweight in lbs ***in kgs***	USDA Min requirement 0.35 g/lb 0.77 g/kg	Physically active requirement 0.52 g/lb 1.13 g/kg	Top level sport requirement 0.68 g/lb 1.5 g/kg
140lbs ***63.6kg***	**49 g**	**72.1 g**	**95.2 g**
<u>160lbs</u> ***72.7kg***	**<u>56 g</u>**	**<u>82.4 g</u>**	**108.8 g**
180lbs ***81.8kg***	**63 g**	**92.7 g**	**122.4 g**
200lbs ***90.9kg***	**70 g**	**110 g**	**136 g**
220lbs **100kg**	**77 g**	**113.3 g**	**149.6 g**
240lbs ***109.1kg***	**84 g**	**123.6 g**	**163.2 g**

Table 16 Activity and Protein Requirement Chart

Okay, so I'm not 40, but we cover the issue of age in more detail in the following Chapter. Just for now we can use this to illustrate the point.

Rather than just estimating my protein requirement as 15% of my total calories, I was looking to estimate the "weight of protein" I needed relative to my bodyweight, which just happens to be 160 lbs. Some days I may be a little less and other days a little more.

And I was taking into account my level of activity each day.

On some days my activity was probably what could be considered average, so I could use the USDA Minimum Requirement Figure. But my active days were certainly not as vigorous as Toby's elite athletes, so I estimated a mid-point which I refer to as "Physically Active".

Using Table 16 above, the estimated protein requirement on my quieter days was 56 g and on my more active days it was 82.4 g. My daily protein requirements for the week are shown on Table 17 below, together with my "Daily Average over the Week".

Day	Activity	Activity Level	Daily Protein
Monday	Work + Strength w/o	Physically Active	82.4 g
Tuesday	Work + General Stuff	Average	56 g
Wednesday	Work + Strength w/o	Physically Active	82.4 g
Thursday	Work + General Stuff	Average	56 g
Friday	Work + Strength w/o	Physically Active	82.4 g
Saturday	Big Run + Family Stuff	Physically Active	82.4 g
Sunday	Recovery Run + Fam Stuff	Physically Active	82.4 g
Daily Average over the Week			**74.8 g**

Table 17 Estimated Activity Levels and Daily Protein

And using this approach I made a rather surprising observation:

My daily protein requirement doesn't change very much.

This becomes more apparent when we take into account how much we actually digest and use from any particular food which we come to shortly.

Furthermore, we can all average our requirements over a few days. A bit more one day and a bit less another is fine. So rather than trying to make an estimate for each day, we can determine our activity levels over several days and determine an average. Then we simply aim to maintain an intake close to this average figure each day.

I found that averaging the calculation of my Proteins over a whole week worked well for me, especially because it made meal planning so much easier. But I appreciate lifestyle or work commitments may require you to use a different timeframe.

And this leads us to what I will call The Calorie Conundrum,

The Calorie Conundrum

I have used a typical week to demonstrate how:

> **My total daily calorie count can fluctuate significantly, but the change to my protein requirement is more modest and can be averaged out over several days.**

I was no longer trying to determine my protein intake on a day-to-day basis. Tuesdays and Thursdays may be my "Rest Days", but the recovery process is still working. I still need my proteins on these days.

So, I was estimating my protein requirements over a whole week based on my overall activity level, then using the average figure each day.

But with my "energy foods", we know from Chapter 8 that we need to top up our energy up on a regular basis. And our "Glucose Battery" for short term energy needs to be topped up through the day.

So, the Calorie Conundrum can be summarized as follows:

- I calculate my Proteins based on a weekly average requirement.
- I calculate my Energy Calories based on a daily requirement.

This disparity is illustrated in the sketched graph in **Fig 7** below. And it really is a sketch because it is just a pattern of eating that I find works for me. We all need to experiment to find what works for our individual lifestyles.

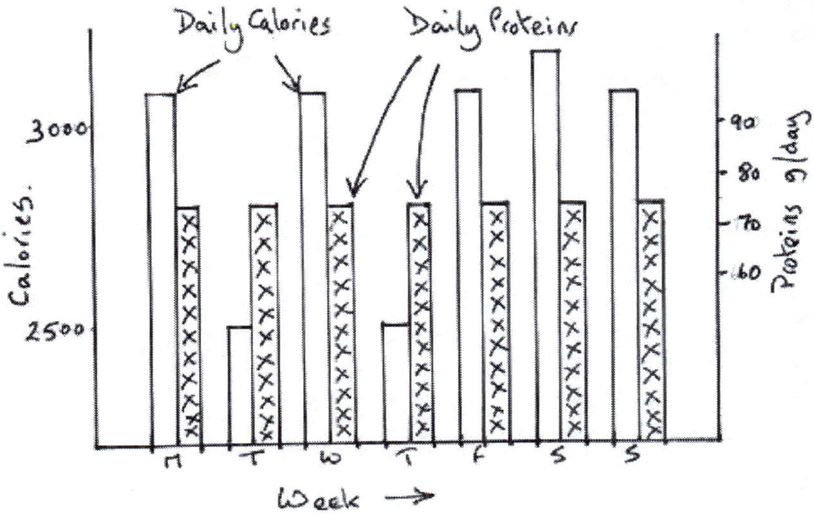

Fig 7. The Calorie Conundrum

And as we experiment and explore our proteins in more detail it is clear that we can all make a good estimation of our genuine daily protein requirement averaged out over a week or whatever timeframe suits you. And this estimation can take into account relevant factors including our bodyweight and activity level.

Replace the Calorie Count with the Protein Count

In the following Chapter we take this a stage further as we explore how to measure or count the proteins in the specific foods we each choose to eat. I suggest that this simple strategy will help you view your food in a completely different way.

I also hope to demonstrate that estimating our proteins is actually quite simple, albeit a bit time consuming at first. But as we progress it is this protein count that will be the key macronutrient measure we use to start planning our daily diet and our meals.

The calorie count is still a useful tool for us. But we will use it to monitor and measure our diet **AFTER** we have included our proteins and all our vitamins, minerals, soluble & insoluble fibres, antioxidants & phytochemicals and probiotics & prebiotics, rather than using it to try and plan all our macronutrients in advance.

In the fullness of time, you might find, as I did, that getting the right amount of my energy foods, my Carbs and Fats, just fell into place.

On more active days I would just include a moderately bigger portion of potato, or rice, or pasta, or legume, whatever my concentrated Carb Food Choice might be.

I even found that after a while I was eating my foods in a loose order. I would eat my proteins and non-starchy veggies before I ate my concentrated Carb Foods.

You might also find, just as I did, that because the protein foods and the fibre rich non-starchy veggies are generally satiating, that it was difficult to eat "too much energy" anyway. In fact, I found that over time the amount of concentrated Carb Foods I needed to include or even just felt like including each day dropped quite dramatically and has stayed that way.

And I should add that I would eat any fruit separately, usually when I felt a bit hungry between meals. I'll explain more in Chapters 29 & 30.

So, this simple switch to Counting Proteins enables us to escape the calorie conundrum and it makes meal planning so much easier. After using the Protein Count to plan, we can use the Calorie Count as the versatile tool it should be to monitor our overall diet making sure we are covering all our nutritional requirements.

So, if we are going to…

Replace Calorie Count with Protein Count

…then we need to look at the Protein Count in more detail.

27. A fresh look at Counting our Proteins

I do appreciate that some vegetarians and vegans can be cautious about proteins. But this affects all of us because:

> **"Regardless of our own individual food preferences, omnivore, carnivore, pescatarian, vegetarian or vegan, we all need the full range of amino acids in our regular diet."**

Just for now we need to put aside all discussions on the rights and wrongs, merits or otherwise of different food preferences and consider how we can each satisfy our own personal requirements for the full range of amino acids from our own food choices.

Remember, we are working with the 20 amino acids of the standard genetic code, and these are listed again in Table 2 on the following page.

We start by looking at what we mean by the terms "Complete" and "High Quality" Proteins and how the body utilizes the constituent Amino Acids.

"Complete" or "High Quality" Proteins

Two terms **"Complete"** and **"High Quality"** can both be used to describe food containing the **full range** of our Essential Amino Acids in roughly **the proportions** that the human body utilizes them.

This is very important because this combination and ratio of amino acids determines how efficiently our bodies absorb and utilize the Proteins from different foods.

Of the two, **I prefer to use the term "Complete"** as I feel this conveys a clearer meaning, so that is what I will use throughout the book.

Essential Amino Acids	Non-Essential Amino Acids
• Histidine	• Alanine
• Isoleucine	• Arginine*
• Leucine	• Asparagine
• Lysine	• Aspartic Acid
• Methionine	• Cysteine
• Phenylalanine	• Glutamic Acid
• Threonine	• Glutamine
• Tryptophan	• Glycine
• Valine	• Proline
	• Serine
	• Tyrosine

Table 2 (Repeat) – Essential and Non-Essential Amino Acids
**Arginine is an Essential Amino Acid for children, but the adult body can synthesize this Amino Acid*

Many of the foods in the "Meat, Fish & Egg" and "Milk & Dairy" Groups contain "Complete" proteins, in other words, all 9 Essential Amino Acids in roughly the proportions that we humans use them.

However, only a modest range of plant-based protein foods contain "Complete" Proteins including:

- Quinoa
- Soy
- Spirulina
- Buckwheat

So, for people who include foods from the "Meat, Fish & Eggs" and, or "Milk & Dairy" food groups in their regular diet, it is relatively easy to include and digest the full range of Essential Amino Acids in roughly the right proportions.

This is also true for any vegetarians who regularly include "Milk & Dairy" foods and possibly even "Eggs" in their diet.

For anyone following a plant-based diet, namely vegans or stricter vegetarians, this can be a challenge because most plant-based protein foods do not contain this "Complete" combination of amino acids.

So, what happens when the foods we eat do not contain the full range of amino acids? What impact does this have on the capacity of the body to digest and absorb the amino acids?

The Biological Value of Protein Foods

Different techniques have been developed to try and measure how much of the total protein content of any given food we are likely to absorb.

One technique gives us a measure called the **Biological Value (BV).** Whilst it does have some limitations it is a simple concept to grasp and as such is a very useful tool for us to use.

The results may be presented using either "percentage utilization" or "relative utilization" protocols. We will use the **"percentage utilization",** in other words the percentage of proteins in the specific foods that are likely to be digested and absorbed.

Table 18 on the following page lists the **amount of protein** contained in some typical food portions, the **biological value of the foods** and then **how much of that protein we are likely to absorb** as "percentage utilization".

We can use these figures to estimate how much protein we are likely to absorb from regular sized portions of these foods. And we will use this Table when we discuss Diet Hack 2 in Chapter 33.

There are other factors that affect the Biological Value such as the Digestive Coefficient, but here we focus on the combination of amino acids.

Protein Food	Typical Portion	Gram of Protein /typical portion	Estimated Biological Value %	Gram of Protein actually absorbed
Whey Protein	30g scoop	20g	98	**19.6g**
Eggs	2 med size	12g	93.7	**11.2g**
Buckwheat	60g ½ cup	11.5g	90	**10.4g**
Milk	240g glass	8g	84.5	**6.8g**
Yoghurt	125g 1 cup	13g	84	**10.9g**
Cheese	2 oz/56.7g	14g	84	**11.8g**
Quinoa	85g ½ cup	11g	83	**9.1g**
Whole Grain Rice	82g ½ cup	3.3g	83	**2.7g**
Fish, salmon	3 oz/85.05g	23g	76	**17.5g**
Seafood, crab	3 oz/85.05g	17g	76	**12.9g**
Beef, rump steak	3 oz/85.05g	26g	74.3	**19.3g**
Chicken, breast	3 oz/85.05g	25g	74	**18.5g**
Tofu firm	3 oz/85.05g	14.5g	74	**10.7g**
Soya Beans, boiled	85g ½ cup	15g	72.8	**10.9g**
Mushrooms	3 oz/85.05g	3g	70	**2.1g**
Quorn	100g	12g	70	**8.4g**
Seeds, sunflower	36g ¼ cup	8g	70	**5.6g**
Legumes, chickpeas	82g ½ cup	8g	68	**5.4g**
Breakfast Cereals	28g 1 cup	2g	*Est (65)	**(1.3g)**
Whole Grain Bread	92g 2 slices	8g	64	**5.1g**
Tree Nuts, pecan	36g ¼ cup	5g	60	**3g**
Beans, dry	85g ½ cup	8g	58	**4.6g**
Lentils	90g half cup	9g	45	**4g**

TABLE 18 The Biological Value of Protein foods

The foods in Table 18 provide a small sample but do illustrate three broad trends:

Foods in the "Meat, Fish & Eggs" and "Milk & Dairy" food groups generally have higher total protein contents than plant foods.

Foods in the "Meat, Fish & Eggs" and "Milk & Dairy" food groups generally have higher Biological Values compared to plant foods.

There are a limited number of notable exceptions including Buckwheat, Quinoa and Soya Beans.

If you recall, "Complete proteins" contain all the Essential Amino Acids and do so in roughly the same proportions as the human body. So, a protein food with a relatively low Biological Value might:

- Be missing one or more of the Essential Amino Acids
- Have very high levels of some and very low levels of others
- Have a combination of both the above

As a result, a lower percentage of protein, or constituent Amino Acids, in the food is digested and absorbed.

Complementary Proteins for Vegans and Vegetarians

As you can see from Table 16, the plant-based proteins like Tree Nuts, Beans and Lentils have relatively low Biological Values. They may be missing or have low values of certain Essential Amino Acids.

But it is possible to achieve more "Complete proteins" by combining different complementary plant proteins. It just takes a little care and planning.

There are numerous excellent sources advising how to achieve this, so for any vegetarians or vegans, you may already have your preferred sites. If not, then just pop in a phrase like "combining plant foods for complete proteins" into your favourite search engine. This is an important issue that is well covered on numerous reputable websites.

The important point is that regardless of our food preferences we can all include all our Essential and Non-Essential Amino Acids in our regular diet through our food choices.

And this brings us to the question, how much "Protein" do we actually need?

The Recommended Daily Allowance and Reference Protein

The Institute of Medicine of the National Academies (United States) developed a measure, their Recommended Daily Allowance (RDA) for Protein which may also be called the Reference Protein. We can describe the two definitions as follows:

Recommended Daily Allowance or RDA

This is calculated and periodically updated by the US Department of Agriculture (USDA) from combined US and Canadian research. The RDA is often quoted using the following example, which is handy for me because my ideal weight is 160 lb give or take a couple of pounds.:

> The USDA recommends 56 grams of protein a day for a 40-year-old man weighing 160 lb and 46 grams of protein for women based on a 40-year-old woman who weighs 140 lb.
>
> That equates to 0.33-0.35 grams of protein for every pound of body weight, or 0.72-0.77 g/kg.

These are the requirements for adults just going about their daily lives. Surprisingly low figures perhaps, but the human body uses proteins very efficiently.

I have deliberately used this example because I find so many sources, especially online, present the following figures as a general guide for all men and women respectively:

- 56 grams of protein for men
- 46 grams of protein for women

BEWARE – Because the example also states:

> "That equates to 0.33-0.35 grams of protein for every pound of body weight, or 0.72-0.77 g/kg."

So, when we are calculating our personal RDA, we also need to account for both gender and variations in bodyweight.

The National Research Council (US) also provide updated guidelines, and these are available online, to download or in print, **(Online Source 32)**. Again, the calculations are updated periodically so you may find sources showing the RDAs with slightly different figures from those above. But don't worry, the differences are minimal, so we can use these figures for our purposes.

Reference Protein and the Reference Nutrient Intake

But as noted back on page 135 and illustrated in Table 18, we do not absorb and digest all the Proteins in our food. Which leads us into a bit of a terminology jumble. So, let's just explore this jumble so we can move forward with confidence.

The term "Reference Nutrient Intake for Protein" is used by The Department of Health here in the UK, in their publication titled "Dietary Reference Values – A Guide published online and available as a PDF Download **(Online Source 33),** and the term can be described as follows:

> This is the level of "Complete Proteins" that each individual needs to **digest and absorb** each day just going about their daily lives.

The term "Reference Protein" can also be used to mean the same thing.

But it can also be used to define one specific Protein source to be used as a standard against which others are measured. For example, egg is often used as a "Reference Protein" in this way.

This interchange of definitions can be confusing, so I was searching for a phrase or term that provided clarity.

Now the National Research Council (US) in their updated guidelines referred to above, also use the term" Reference Proteins", but in a specific way. They refer to the:

"RDA of Reference Proteins"

Now I find this term provides the clarity I am after, and I have adopted and used term to mean:

> The level of "Complete Proteins" that each individual needs to **digest and absorb** each day as we are just going about our daily lives.

This then highlights a question:

> If this is the amount we need just going about our daily lives, should we treat this as our "Minimum Protein Requirement"?

I will go on to explain why and how I use the calculation of my "RDA of Reference Proteins" as the minimum target I should include each day.

But before we explore this issue further, we need to re-visit the issue of how much protein we can absorb and digest from our different Protein Foods.

The RDA of Reference Proteins and Biological Values of Food

On page 135 we discussed the Biological Value (BV) of foods and how this affects how much protein we can absorb and digest from different foods.

Table 18 highlights how the BV varies significantly with examples of 93.7% for eggs and 45% for lentils. But this is not the whole picture because foods, or specifically plant-based foods can be combined to increase the overall BV of the combined proteins.

So, regardless of the source of my proteins, I need to determine the amount of Protein I need to include in my food in order to absorb and digest my "RDA of Reference Proteins". And I need to allow for variations in uptake from different foods, depending on their Biological Value.

We cover this aspect in detail in Chapter 33 but first we need to clarify how we can all make a reasonable estimate of our genuine "RDA of Reference Proteins".

RDA of Reference Proteins by Weight and Activity Levels

Now we can take the RDA example on page 138 and on page 139 note that calculating our individual requirements:

> Equates to 0.33-0.35 grams of protein for every pound of body weight, or 0.72-0.77 g/kg.

And that these protein levels are for 40-year-old adults:

> Just going about their daily lives

We will come back to the issue of age shortly, but first we need to address variation in bodyweight and variation in activity level.

> **Bodyweight** - For two people living a similar lifestyle it seems to make sense that a person with a larger physical stature requires more energy and more protein than another with a naturally lighter build.
>
> But when we consider our bodyweight, we should be using a reasonable estimate of our ideal weight. So, if we know that we are 20-30 lbs overweight then we don't need to add extra proteins (or energy) for that excess weight.
>
> Conversely, when I was seriously ill, I was also seriously underweight, in other words well below my ideal weight. So, I needed to add more proteins as I rebuilt my health and fitness.
>
> **Activity Level** - Back in Chapter 26 we addressed how our daily calorie requirement increases as we become more active and how the increase in proteins may best be estimated by weight. I used the example of the GB Rowing Squad recommending an increased Protein intake by weight for their athletes involved in a very intensive training regime.

Now we can bring these two factors together and illustrate this by comparing two sets of estimated proteins requirements. These are for males and females both aged 40 across a range of bodyweights and different activity levels, as shown in Table 16 repeated below.

Protein Requirement for Female aged 40			
Bodyweight in lbs. ***in kgs***	**1** USDA Min requirement 0.33 g/lb. 0.72 g/kg	**2** Physically active requirement 0.51 g/lb. 1.12 g/kg	**3** Top level sport requirement 0.68 g/lb. 1.5 g/kg
100lbs ***45.5kg***	**33 g**	**50.5 g**	**68 g**
<u>120lbs</u> ***54.5kg***	**<u>39.6 g</u>**	**<u>60.6 g</u>**	**81.6 g**
140lbs ***63.6kg***	**46.2 g**	**70.7 g**	**95.2 g**
160lbs ***72.7kg***	**52.8 g**	**80.8 g**	**108.8 g**
180lbs ***81.8kg***	**59.4 g**	**90.9 g**	**122.4 g**
200lbs ***90.6kg***	**66 g**	**101 g**	**136 g**
Protein Requirement for Male aged 40			
Bodyweight in lbs. ***in kgs***	USDA Min requirement 0.35 g/lb. 0.77 g/kg	Physically active requirement 0.52 g/lb. 1.13 g/kg	Top level sport requirement 0.68 g/lb. 1.5 g/kg
140lbs ***63.6kg***	**49 g**	**72.1 g**	**95.2 g**
<u>160lbs</u> ***72.7kg***	**<u>56 g</u>**	**<u>82.4 g</u>**	**108.8 g**
180lbs ***81.8kg***	**63 g**	**92.7 g**	**122.4 g**
200lbs ***90.9kg***	**70 g**	**110 g**	**136 g**
220lbs **100kg**	**77 g**	**113.3 g**	**149.6 g**
240lbs ***109.1kg***	**84 g**	**123.6 g**	**163.2 g**

Table 16 (Repeat) - Activity and Protein Requirement Chart

Column 1 shows the estimated RDA of Reference Proteins based on the subjects just going about their daily lives.

- Females – 0.33 g per lb of Bodyweight (or 0.72 g per kg of Bodyweight)
- Males – 0.35 g per lb of Bodyweight (or 0.77 g per kg of Bodyweight)

Column 3 shows the estimated RDA of Reference Proteins for a very high level of activity. In this example the athletes are engaged in intense training to International Rowing Standards.

- Females – 0.68 g per lb of Bodyweight (or 1.5 g per kg of Bodyweight)
- Males – 0.68 g per lb of Bodyweight (or 1.5 g per kg of Bodyweight)

Column 2 shows the estimated RDA of Reference Proteins I use for my personal requirements on days when I am physically active.

Now I am not active or training to the same level as International Rowers, but my own sessions may include running over 4-9 miles, ergo sessions, heavy weights, body circuits and Kettlebells.

So, I can make a good estimate of where I sit between the ends of the Activity Spectrum and so I use the following:

- Males – 0.52 g per lb of Bodyweight (or 1.13 g per kg of Bodyweight)
- Females – 0.51 g per lb of Bodyweight (or 1.12 g per kg of Bodyweight)

The three data sets illustrate that the amounts of "RDA of Reference Proteins" we need are surprisingly modest, highlighting again just how efficiently the body utilizes the amino acids.

And I stress you should also use your "ideal bodyweight". If you know you are 20-30 lbs. over, those extra pounds do not need extra proteins.

And conversely, if you are 10-20 lbs. under, then add a bit more to help you attain your ideal bodyweight, if that is what you want to do.

RDA of Reference Proteins Averaged out over a Week

In the previous Chapter describing the Calorie Conundrum I explained how it is useful to estimate our activity level over a few days and preferentially over a week.

Of course, our activity levels can fluctuate through the week. In my own case I used an example when my typical week included five days when I was "Physically Active" and two "Average Days".

Through the course of the year and from year to year this might change. But it is very easy to revise this figure for any given week.

I plan my exercise and activities by the week, so I have just found this weekly estimate the easiest to use. You may use a different timeframe.

It certainly makes meal planning much easier, as I cover in due course.

Too Much or Too Little Protein?

The levels for the "RDA of Reference Proteins" in Table 16 are indeed modest and are often countered with warnings that eating too much protein can cause serious health issues. So, how can we make sense of these figures?

The first point to bear in mind is that the levels in Column 1 of the Table are the minimum requirements, not some sort of healthy average or optimal figure. So:

> A 140lb woman leading a relatively quiet life needs to digest and absorb a minimum 46.2g of "Complete Proteins" to
>
> - retain all the key functions controlled by proteins
> - and maintain her skeletal muscle mass.

If this level is **the minimum requirement** this raises some interesting questions:

1. Are we potentially compromising our health if we fail to meet these minimum requirements?

2. Should this be increased to achieve an adequate or better still an optimal level?

Using the example of the rowing athletes training to international level

> The equivalent woman engaged in high level sport, or a very active lifestyle needs a minimum of 95.2g of digested and absorbed reference proteins.

In much the same way that there are all sorts of messages urging us to "Eat Low Fat" or "No Fat" Diets, I also appreciate that there seem to be all sorts of messages warning about "Eating Too Much Protein".

So, we must explore this issue to make sure we aren't compounding a potential health issue. And we start by examining the methodology for measuring our Protein requirements.

How accurate is the method for measuring the RDA of Protein?

As with many measurements, it is not possible to actually measure the protein directly. Rather the levels of Nitrogen are measured and the relationship to the Proteins inferred.

In their book *"The Sacred Cow"*, **(Ref 12)** authors Diana Rodgers and Robb Wolf provide an interesting quote from the report defining the Reference Proteins, which reads as follows:

> *"In adults, it is generally presumed that the protein requirement is achieved when an individual is in zero nitrogen balance. To some extent, this assumption poses problems that may lead to underestimates of the true protein requirement."*

Diana Rodgers and Robb Wolf go on to point out that these Reference Protein Figures are a minimum. Furthermore, the Institute of Medicine of the National Academies (United States), provide a different approach in which the recommended Protein intake is between 10 and 30% of the total calorie intake. This is referred to as the Acceptable Macronutrient Distribution Range or the AMDR,

This would set an upper limit equivalent to 1.36 g per lb of Bodyweight (or 3 g per kg of Bodyweight). This is twice the level set for the High-Level Athletes in Table 16.

This upper limit is considerably higher than most sources recommend. So, does eating this amount risk causing any health problems? This in turn raises another question:

How much is too much Protein?

Diana Roberts and Robb Wolf go on to explain that there is no evidence that protein levels of up to 3g per kg of bodyweight pose any health risks.

But that doesn't mean that they recommend eating such high levels. Reading their book, I would say their main concern is to make sure that.

> ...people are not so alarmed at possible health risks associated with supposedly high levels of protein that they then inadvertently aim too low with the opposite risk to their health, too little protein.

In his book, *"How Much Protein"*, **(Ref 4)** Brad Pilon explores the question in terms of how much protein is required to support healthy muscle mass and makes the following observation:

> *"However, there has been research published that suggests that the current RDA for protein (0.36 grams per pound bodyweight) may be inadequate for the maintenance of skeletal muscle in older adults [Campbell, WW 1994], and this book does agree with the idea that intakes higher than the RDA seem to be involved in a better (or at least faster) response to muscle building. The range of 70-120 grams of protein is typically above 0.5 grams protein per pound of bodyweight for most individuals, and would be classified as 'high protein' in the scientific world."*

And please note, the reference to RDA for protein of 0.36grams per pound of bodyweight is a direct comparison with the Reference Protein of 0.35g in Table 16. The figures are adjusted periodically so sources from different dates may vary slightly.

Now we can use his reference to "the range of 70-120 grams of protein is typically above 0.5g per pound of bodyweight" for our own purposes.

This is roughly halfway between the minimum RDA of Reference Protein measure of 0.36 grams and the 0.68g recommended by British Rowing for the Top-Level Athletes. And this just happens to equate to the figure I was using and continue to use for myself.

Brad Pilon also makes the point that the RDA of proteins can be averaged out over a few days.

And he eloquently describes how the amino acids are quite literally like little building blocks that can be shuffled around the body to wherever they are needed and then on to somewhere else in due course.

So, it seems that the range of Protein Intakes in Table 16 gives us a good baseline to cover our minimum requirements and we have some latitude to increase this a bit as we each strive to define an adequate level or better still an optimal level of protein in our own diet?

Taking Age into Account

We have considered the implications of gender, bodyweight and activity level, so now we can address the issue of age.

As I said right at the start, the book has specifically been written for adults. The issue of diet for young children and teenagers are specialist areas again. My wife and I did use the general principles of the 3 Diet Hacks with our own children but that was our personal choice. And we tried to take into consideration some of the advice from specialist books and websites to provide an optimum level of protein through their growing years.

At the other end of the age spectrum, as we get on in years, we can all experience the issue of muscle loss and a less efficient capacity to utilize our dietary proteins. Unfortunately, the lost muscle mass may be replaced by increased body fat.

I maintain the same weight and nearly the same muscle mass by including strength training in my weekly routines and eating a bit more protein again to compensate for the decreased efficiency in utilizing the proteins from my diet.

I'm not trying to fight the effects of aging and chase eternal youth, I just enjoy keeping strong, fit and healthy. And I can make sure that I do have enough Protein in my diet by including a bit more without any sort of risk to my health and enough to feel confident that I have covered all my amino acids to stay healthy.

Getting All Our Amino Acids

This is an opportune time to remind ourselves that it is the constituent Amino Acids in our Protein Foods that the body needs, as we discovered back in Chapter 9.

Furthermore, it does not matter what your food preferences are, or your age, weight or activity level:

We all need ALL our Amino Acids

In fact, I would suggest that including all our Amino Acids in our regular diet and in sufficient quantities is just as important as including all our vitamins and all our minerals.

Striving for an Optimal Protein intake in our Diet

It is important to understand that the intention here is not to regulate our daily proteins down to fractions of a gram. That would be futile and take a lot of time.

My intention is to highlight the importance of proteins in our daily nutrition across all the possible food preferences and choices.

The issues covered here raise a number of interesting points and possible questions:

1. The level of RDA of Reference Proteins refers to the amount of Protein, or rather Amino Acids, that are **digested and absorbed** for the body to use.

2. Should we treat the level of RDA of Reference Proteins as the **minimum required** to maintain all the key functions controlled by Proteins in the body?
3. If we fail to meet the level of RDA of Reference Proteins on a regular basis could this have **health repercussions** in the same way as failing to meet the full daily Vitamin or Mineral requirements?
4. Can we include **a bit more Protein** in the daily diet without any serious health repercussions?

Of course, I am not offering health advice here. I am merely presenting the evidence that I used to make my own choices. I felt confident that it was better to have a bit more Protein than I calculated as my minimum without worrying about any adverse health risks.

There are so many ways we can each meet our protein requirements regardless of our food preferences. So, I want to encourage you to explore your options safe in the knowledge that you are including sufficient proteins to maintain your full health and not putting your health at risk if you eat a bit too much.

We can all experiment to find our own optimal protein level by "Counting our Proteins".

Indeed, this aspect of your diet is so important that Diet Hack 2 is all about "Counting your Proteins" and shows you how to:

- Make a reasonable estimate of your daily protein intake based on your gender, optimal bodyweight and activity level.
- Include a variety and range of protein foods in your diet to cover all your amino acids.
- Use the Biological Value of Foods to make sure to digest and absorb sufficient protein and to strive to achieve the optimal Protein intake in your regular diet.

A Surprising Outcome

There is one more surprising outcome or benefit to this approach.

In my own experience, I found by using the 3 Diet Hacks sequentially, in other words including my "5 a Day", then "Counting my Proteins", my Carbs and Fats seemed to fall into place quite easily.

It reminds me of the quote from Balz Frei, Emeritus Professor at Oregon State University, back on Page 89:

> *Research indicates that the body is well adapted to utilize the micronutrients in fresh produce, just taking what it needs.*

My own observation was that after eating all my non-starchy veggies, fruit and proteins, I seemed to find a happy balance with my Carbs and Fats without any real effort. But maybe that's just me.

I want to finish this chapter by encouraging you to explore the different foods that suit your preferences, tastes and budget and strive to find your optimal level of protein.

And I also want you to enjoy your food. Your diet should be an adventure not some rigid sufferance. Which leads us rather appropriately to our Fats.

28. Good Fats, Bad Fats

We need our Fats and yet the Fats are probably the most controversial of all our Food Types and possibly the most maligned.

In Chapter 10 we explored four of the polyunsaturated fats that are classified as Essential Nutrients. But I also highlighted that we need a variety of other fats in our diet, and we need them for a host of reasons including the following:

- Fats are a primary source for our energy.
- A number of our vitamins are fat soluble.
- Fats are building blocks of key hormones such as Testosterone, Human Growth Hormone and Estrogen.
- The balance between dietary fats and carbs is essential for optimal energy production.

The Fats are an important Food Type and one of our three macronutrients. To help us explore the different Fats we can categorize them into four main sub types as follows:

- Saturated Fats
- Polyunsaturated Fats including the Omega 3 and Omega 6 Fatty Acids
- Monosaturated Fats including the Omega 9 Fatty Acids
- Trans Fats and Hydrogenated Oils

Saturated Fats – or SFAs

These are the main fats usually associated with Meat and Dairy foods and they are generally thoroughly maligned. Indeed, many sources suggest removing them from our diet altogether. But there is more to them than this characterization might suggest. Let's start by exploring the full range of these Fats.

The Saturated Fats are identified by the length of the carbon chain as shown in Table 19 opposite. While these may be divided into four further sub-categories, for now we will focus on the following three:

> **Long Chain Fatty Acids** – Stearic Acid and Palmitic Acid are associated with Meat and most Dairy Foods, apart from Goat's Milk. Whilst we might immediately think of these as problematic, especially in terms of bad cholesterol, they are each quite different as we cover shortly.
>
> The third of these, Myristic Acid, is found in the milk of Cows, Sheep and Buffalo, but not Goat. This Fat raises the levels of LDL (bad) cholesterol but is usually only found in small amounts.
>
> **Medium Chain Fatty Acids** – Three of the four, Lauric, Capric and Caprylic Acid, are found in Goat's Milk and indeed the very names of the latter two are derived from the Latin for female goat, Capra.
>
> The fourth, Caproic Acid is found in other Dairy foods from Cows, Sheep and Buffalo.
>
> But this category is also found in a range of plant foods. When these Fats occur in foods like Coconut Oil they may be referred to as Medium Chain Triglycerides or MCTs. These Fats are considered healthy because they are readily absorbed in the digestive system and transported to the liver where they are also readily metabolized.
>
> **Short Chain Fatty Acids** – These are only found in very minor amounts, if any, in the food we eat. However, when our good bacteria ferment our Prebiotic Fibres in the large

intestine, the process can produce these Saturated Fats. They are readily absorbed and utilized for energy.

Common Name	Length of Carbon Chain	Main Animal Foods
Very Long Chain Fatty Acids		
Lignoceric Acid	24	
Behenic Acid	22	
Long Chain Fatty Acids		
Arachidic Acid	20	Fish
Stearic Acid	18	Meat Dairy& Fish
Palmitic Acid	16	Meat Dairy & Fish
Myristic Acid	14	Dairy
Medium Chain Fatty Acids		
Lauric Acid	12	Goats Milk
Capric Acid	10	
Caprylic Acid	8	
Caproic Acid	6	Dairy
Short Chain Fatty Acids		
Butyric Acid	4	Dairy & Fish g
Propionic Acid	3	
Acetic Acid	2	Vinegar

Table 19 Our Saturated Fats

It seems that nothing is straight forward with our Saturated Fats. So, when we consider the health risks of Saturated Fats especially with regard to cholesterol, we do find a couple of strange pairings, as follows:

Stearic Acid and Palmitic Acid - Stearic Acid is the second most common saturated fat in the American Diet. This might sound like bad news, but it may lower the levels of LDL (bad) cholesterol.

However, Palmitic Acid is the most common saturated fat in the American diet, and it not only raises the level of overall cholesterol but may increase the level of LDL (bad) cholesterol.

And yet at the same time, Palmitic Acid is the most common Saturated Fat found in the human body and the body even has the capacity to synthesize this Saturated Fat.

Myristic Acid and Lauric Acid – Now these both raise blood cholesterol. But the former raises the overall level of cholesterol and in particular the LDL (bad) cholesterol, whereas the latter increases the level of HDL (good) cholesterol.

And it gets more complicated when we start to appreciate that the Saturated Fats are also found in all sorts of plant foods. We have already mentioned the Medium Chain Triglycerides (MCTs) in Coconut, plus of course Palmitic Acid which even derives the name from Palm Oil.

It turns out that Saturated Fats are found in a host of plant foods but usually in smaller amounts than found in Meat and Dairy Foods.

Whilst we hear a lot about the bad aspects of saturated fats, we must also bear in mind that we do need them in moderation as outlined by Atli Arnarson in his article titled "10 Types of Saturated Fats Reviewed" published online, **(Online Source 34).** It seems that they can be part of our diet in moderation, but we must treat these with some caution.

Polyunsaturated Fats – or PUFAs

Whilst we should treat our Saturated Fats with a bit of caution, the Polyunsaturated Fats are quite the opposite it seems. These Fats provide all sorts of benefits, and they are the only Fats regarded as Essential in our diet and there are two main categories as follows:

Omega 3 Fatty Acids – This category includes some 11 different Fats, but only three are considered Essential and these are:

- Alpha-linolenic acid or ALA
- Eicosapentaenoic Acid or EPA
- Docosahexaenoic Acid or DHA

ALA is the parent fatty acid of the Omega 3 family, and this family of fatty acids plays an important role in a range of functions. We come back to the specific functions of EPA & DHA shortly, but the parent ALA is considered to have a beneficial effect on functions including:

- Reducing Triglyceride in the blood
- Reducing irregular heart rhythms
- Slowing the build-up of plaque in arteries
- Slightly reducing blood pressure

Omega 6 Fatty Acids – This category includes 4 different Fats but only one is considered Essential and this is:

- Linoleic Acid or LA

Like ALA and the omega 3s, LA is the parent fatty acid of the Omega 6s and this is the one we will focus on here.

LA is considered to have a beneficial effect on functions including:

- Controlling your blood sugar
- Reducing your risk for diabetes
- Lowering your blood pressure

And it is important to stress that I am not trying to offer medical advice here, I am merely reporting benefits widely attributed to these nutrients.

But whilst these health benefits are important, the aspect that sets this sub type of Fats apart is the impact on the human brain.

EPA, DHA, Omega 6, and the Brain

In Chapter 10 we covered how the Long Chain Fatty Acid Omega 3s, EPA and DHA, together with the Omega 6 LA are particularly important for our brains.

It seems that DHA might be particularly important as one of the key contributing factors enabling the creation of the more complex neural networks. The brain capacity resulting from these complex neural networks set modern humans apart. Indeed, they play a fundamental role in making us human in the first place.

Whilst the health benefits of the various Polyunsaturated Fats are widely recognized, we can consider the sources of these Fats and two areas of controversy.

Sources of EPA and DHA – The body does have the capacity to synthesize both EPA and DHA from the parent ALA. This is why some sources do not treat these as Essential Nutrients.

However, there does seem to be considerable doubt that the body can synthesize the full requirement of both Long Chain Fatty Acids on a regular basis.

The main (modern) food source of EPA and DHA are fish based and particularly from oily fish such as Salmon and Sardines. They also usually occur with the parent Omega 3, ALA, and parent Omega 6 LA in these fish-based foods.

As a result, we tend to consider oily fish as the primary natural source in the modern diet. This is why respected organizations such as the Harvard School of Public Health in the USA and the NHS in the UK both recommend that we all include food sources such as Oily fish, such as salmon at least twice a week.

And if this was not possible, they both recommend using supplements to maintain these important nutrients in the regular diet. Many of the supplements are based on either Fish Oil or Krill Oil.

This obviously presents an issue for Vegetarians and Vegans who would not want to eat any Fish or other animal Foods However, other supplements are available based on algae, the original source of EPA and DHA in the diet of both fish and krill.

It is interesting to note that in the not-so-distant past, meat cuts from grass fed cattle and sheep provided significant levels of both EPA and DHA, as highlighted back in Chapter 10 **(Ref 5)**. It is ironic that "modern" livestock farming methods have reduced the amount of these essential nutrients from a regular food source for many. That's progress for you!

Coming back to the recommendation to eat a couple of portions of oily fish or to take supplements, again, I am not offering health advice here, I am merely reporting a recommendation made by two respected authorities on health and nutrition. Always consult your doctor for health advice regarding your diet.

Sources of Omega 3 and Omega 6 – The parent Fatty Acids of both Omega 3s and Omega 6 Fats, ALA and LA are both found in many plant-based foods. These include:

- **Grains** like Corn and Oats
- **Tree Nuts** like Walnut
- **Seeds** like Safflower, Rapeseed, Flaxseed, Hempseeds
- **Legumes** like Soybean, Chickpeas, Peanuts
- **Fruit** like Avocado

This all sounds like excellent news. We all have many food choices we can call upon for these important nutrients. But there may be a catch.

Excess Omega 6 in the diet -The ready availability of the parent Fatty Acids of both Omega 3s and Omega 6 Fats, is all very encouraging except for one thing. We humans should have a balance of Omega 6 to Omega 3 in the range between 1-to-1 and 4-to1.

But we humans are introducing new foods like concentrated Seed oils into the diet, and these may be very high in Omega 6. This in turn is pushing the ratio of Omega 6 to Omega 3 well over 15-to-1 and there is concern that this is creating a new health issue.

A P Simopoulos outlines this issue in his paper titled "The importance of the ratio of omega-6 to omega-3 essential fatty acids" published online, **(Online Source 35)**.

It seems our Polyunsaturated Fats are both good for us and potentially bad for us. In particular, the Omega 3s including the Long Chain Fatty Acids and Omega 6s are **essential** for a host of functions.

And I refer you again to the paper titled: "Omega 3 Fatty Acids EPA and DHA: Health Benefits Throughout Life." By Danielle Swanson. Robert Block and Shaker A. Mousa, **(Online Source 6)**.

EPA and DHA are particularly important for our brains. They are an important part of being human.

But conversely new foods rich in Omega 6 may be creating a new health issue as the ratio of Omega 3 to Omega 6 is being affected. It is not clear yet how the excess of Omega 6 may impact on our health, but it is an issue that deserves our attention.

Monounsaturated Fats or MUFAs

These are also referred to as the Omega 9 Fats. Of all the Monounsaturated Fats, Oleic Acid is the most common and the most abundant in most diets.

This is also the main fat the body uses both for energy and to store in the adipose cells.

The Oleic Acid we need can either be synthesized from other fats or it can be ingested directly in our diet which is why it is not considered Essential.

We will focus on this one fat because it is by far the most important Monounsaturated Fat in our diet.

Oleic Acid is generally considered to be a healthy fat and is one of the main Fats found in many plant foods including:

- **Grains** like Rice, Corn and Oats
- **Tree Nuts** like Walnut
- **Seeds** like Grape seed Sunflower, Rapeseed, Hempseeds
- **Legumes** like Chickpeas, Orange Lentil, Pea and Fava Bean
- **Fruit** like Avocado and Olive, although free Oleic Acid renders Olive Oil inedible

It is also found combined with both our saturated fats and polyunsaturated fats in some Meat, Fish and Dairy Foods.

It seems our Monounsaturated Fats, and particularly Oleic Acid, are good for us and should be included in our regular diet. We can appreciate that Oleic Acid in particular, is a key source of energy. However, we still need to monitor how much we include because of course the fats have more than twice as much energy per gram weight as the carbohydrates.

We also need to be aware that our Monounsaturated Fats are usually combined with other types of fats. So, we need to take this into consideration in our food choices.

Trans Fats and Hydrogenated Oils –

The Trans Fats are a form of Unsaturated Fat that may be found in some animal-based foods. They are formed by bacteria in the gut of the animal and may then be present in small amounts in various types of meat or dairy products.

They are regarded as unhealthy but usually only occur in small amounts.

It is the highly processed man-made Trans Fats which really should be treated with care. These are formed during a process called hydrogenation. This process is used to alter the characteristics of liquid unsaturated fats by the addition of hydrogen. This increases the melting point of the fats producing a fat that is solid at room temperature which may be called shortening, or vegetable shortening. The process increases the shelf life of the fat.

Vegetable Shortening made from partially hydrogenated vegetable oil was invented in the early 1900s. It provided a cheap alternative to butter and also offered different cooking characteristics. Pastry cooks will be familiar with the flakier pastry made with these products.

Many food manufacturers will use these fats because they are cheaper than natural products and for the different cooking characteristics they bring. They may help:

- Improve taste.
- Improve texture.
- Increase shelf life.

Unfortunately, these man-made Trans Fats found specifically in the partially hydrogenated oils, are found to both increase levels of LDL (bad) cholesterol and decrease the levels of HDL (good) cholesterol.

We can find the hydrogenated oils and the trans fats they contain in so many processed foods like:

- Vegetable shortenings
- Bakery products like muffins
- Margarines and cooking Oils
- Fast Foods fried in vegetable oils
- Pastry products like pies and pizzas

It seems that the process of hydrogenation can produce a product that both food manufacturers and we the consumers prefer.

However, the resulting hydrogenated oils can contain trans fats with serious health implications as reported by Fred A Kummerow in his paper titled "The negative effects of hydrogenated trans fats and what to do about them" published online, **(Online Source 36).** And there have been some moves to restrict the production of the more harmful hydrogenated oils and remove these from processed foods. But in the end, we should all take steps to avoid these whenever possible.

Identifying Good Fats Bad Fats in our Diet

In Chapters 8 and 26 we discussed the macronutrients and highlighted how the Fats should make up something like 35% of our daily calories. For a range of 2000 -2500 calories per day, this would equate to something like 80-100 grams (2.5 - 3.5 oz) of total fat content of the diet. It seems that we need our Fats.

We also need different Fats but as we explore our foods, we find that the different types and sub types of Fats don't occur in isolation.

There are different saturated Fats in many plant foods, albeit in smaller quantities than in Meats and Dairy Foods. Some plant foods high in Saturated Fats are touted as particularly healthy, such as coconut oil. And it does seem that the body uses some saturated Fats for energy.

We need to understand how the Fats work for us. To help us do this we can identify them as good and bad fats as follows:

> **Monounsaturated Fats** – These are regarded as healthy fats for good reasons.
>
> Fats are one of our three macronutrients, and the most common and abundant Monounsaturated Fat Oleic Acid is also the main fat used by the body both for energy and to store energy.
>
> The body can also synthesize Oleic Acid from other fats and carbohydrates. This is the fat that should make up the bulk of our daily fat intake.

Polyunsaturated Fats – These are essential nutrients and provide a host of health benefits.

We only need them in relatively small amounts compared to our energy needs, but we must all pay attention to include both the parent Omega 3 ALA and Omega 6 LA in our regular diet. These may be found in many plant foods.

We should also include the Long Chain Omega 3s EPA and DHA found in fish and seafood. These foods cause an issue for vegetarians and vegans looking for natural food sources, but algae-based supplements are now available.

Surprisingly, because of the introduction of new foods like "seed oils" from Rapeseed (Canola), Sunflower and other seeds rich in Omega 6, there may be a health issue associated with increased intake of Omega 6 relative to the Omega 3s.

Saturated Fats – It seems that we do need some of these fats in our diet to help balance our hormones.

Some of these, particularly the Medium Chain Fatty Acids found in Dairy Foods and in some plant foods, where they are referred to as MCTs, are also deemed to be healthy.

And curiously the body synthesizes one of the Long Chain Fatty Acids. The Gut Flora may also produce Short Chain Fatty Acids, and these are readily absorbed and used by the body for energy.

But we should treat these with a bit of caution because too much of the wrong Long Chain Saturated Fats typically found in Meat foods may have health implications.

Trans Fats and Hydrogenated Oils – These are the Fats to avoid.

Whilst there are natural Trans Fats found in small quantities in some Meat Foods, it is the man-made Trans Fats we need to be wary of.

They provide a cheap source of versatile fats for all sorts of food production, and they also represent the most harmful of all the fats. And they lend themselves to properties of texture, taste and shelf life which means they are widely used.

Despite this widespread use, they really should be treated with the utmost caution. Ideally, they should be avoided altogether, or at the very least just kept to a minimum.

All we can do is to be aware and find alternatives if we can.

Understanding our Fats is the Key

Our Fats can cause some confusion, but if we choose to understand them and how they meet our nutritional needs then we can start to make informed choices.

We do need Fats in our diet, and we need the different types including Monounsaturated, Polyunsaturated and even our Saturated Fats. Fats work together with the Carbs for efficient energy, they provide the Fat-Soluble Vitamins, specific Fats are essential for our brains and even our cardiovascular health.

In fact, for anyone eating between 2000 -2500 calories per day, Fats should make up something like 35% of those daily calories. This equates to something like 80-100 grams (2.5 - 3.5 oz).

It seems that we do not need to be scared of our fats, even the saturated fats. But it does seem prudent that we should only use seed-based fats or oils with high levels of Omega 6 in moderation and we should try to avoid the man-made Trans Fats altogether.

29. Good Carbs, Bad Carbs

The human body uses a specific type of sugar called glucose as the primary energy source. We obtain the glucose we need directly from foods containing glucose or from other sugars and starches in different foods that either contain glucose or can be converted into glucose. These foods are our Carbohydrates.

Carbohydrates are often classified as either Simple Carbs or Complex Carbs and that appears straight forward enough. But as with everything to do with nutrition these terms can be used to mean different things. Indeed, sometimes the Simple Carbs may be referred to as "Sugars" and because the Sugars form the building blocks of all Carbohydrates, we'll start there.

Sugars or Simple Carbs

The Sugars or Simple Carbs can be classified into two sub types as follows:

Monosaccharides

These are the building blocks of all sugars and indeed of all Carbohydrates, and we are interested in the following three monosaccharides:

- Glucose
- Fructose
- Galactose

The body produces a fourth Monosaccharide, Ribose, but that is beyond the scope of this book as we are interested in the sugars found primarily in our foods.

And Dextrose is a form of Glucose derived particularly from Corn. It is chemically identical to Glucose and the names are often interchanged. We will just use the term Glucose here.

When we eat foods containing Fructose or Galactose, they must be converted to Glucose for the body to be able to use them. They are absorbed in the small intestine then transported to the liver where they can be metabolized to glucose. The liver has a limited capacity to metabolize both fructose and galactose and we come back to these in due course.

Disaccharides

The Monosaccharides are often found in paired combinations and the three main pairs or Disaccharides are:

- **Sucrose** - A combination of Glucose and Fructose that is found in many fruits and vegetables. Sucrose refined from sugar cane or sugar beet is referred to as Table Sugar.

- **Lactose** - A combination of Glucose and Galactose. This is mainly found in Dairy Foods and requires the body to produce the enzyme lactase to break the Lactose down to the constituent sugars. Most babies produce lactase to digest the lactose in breast milk. However, a significant percentage of adults lose the capacity to produce lactase resulting in Lactose Intolerance. This is particularly so for whole populations in Asia and Africa.

- **Maltose** - A combination of Glucose and Glucose. Whilst occurring naturally in some foods like Grains and some Starchy Vegetables, Maltose may also be created when processing foods by fermentation or simply by heating.

Galactose and Lactose are generally associated with Dairy Foods. Whilst Galactose may be found in small amounts in other foods and Maltose in a limited number of foods, we will set these aside for most of our discussion and concentrate on the other Sugars:

Glucose | Sucrose | Fructose

These Sugars or Simple Carbs occur naturally in all sorts of combinations in different foods, particularly our Fruits and Non-Starchy Vegetables. Many of these foods contain a combination of all three and some a combination of two. The Canadian Sugar Institute provides a useful online resource on Sugars including an article titled "Sources of Sugars"**, (Online Source 37).**

There are a few exceptions where the sugar content is almost entirely Sucrose. These include Sugar Cane, Sugar Beet and, strangely enough, Sweet Peas. Both Sugar Cane and Sugar Beet are grown on a large scale for the commercial production of Sucrose or Table Sugar. We will come back to these shortly.

It seems that the Sugars occur naturally in so many foods we would normally regard as healthy, which may come as a surprise. But before we address that we should also note that these Sugars can also occur with Polysaccharides.

Polysaccharides or Complex Carbs

The Polysaccharides or Complex Carbs are all made by joining glucose in different ways and most sources will list three as follows:

- **Starches** - This is the type of complex carbohydrate that the body can digest, though often they require some cooking. The starches are formed from long chains of Glucose molecules which can be straight or branched. These chains can be broken down into the constituent glucose and used by the body for energy.

But there are some starches, referred to as Resistant Starches, that the body cannot break down. We will come back to these shortly.

The Starches are important for our energy requirements and are particularly found in most Grains, Pseudo Cereals and Legumes.

- **Cellulose** – This is the main substance found in plant walls. The cellulose provides the strength and structure of the plant walls. When we include this in our food, we refer to the cellulose as our Insoluble Fibre.

  You will recall that we do not digest these Insoluble Fibres in the same way as sugars, fats or proteins. However, they facilitate a number of key functions in the dietary tract as we covered in Chapter 16 and as such, they are one of our Vital Nutrients

  And some of these fibres feed the good bacteria in the Gut Flora, as described in Chapter 17. These specific fibres are also one of our Vital Nutrients and are referred to as our Prebiotics.

- **Glycogen** – This starch is produced by the body to enable storage of Glucose energy. The glycogen, also called Animal Starch, can then be stored in a number of locations around the body, particularly in the liver and in the skeletal muscles.

There are a few other Polysaccharides which we will loosely group together as:

- **Soluble Fibres** – These include the Resistant Fibres mentioned earlier together with a range of pectins and gums that may be dissolved or partially dissolved in the dietary tract.

  Like the Insoluble fibres, these Soluble Fibres perform key functions in the dietary tract. Some also feed the good bacteria and are also referred to as Prebiotics, as we covered back in Chapters 16 and 17.

Untangling Simple and Complex Carbs

The Simple and Complex Carbs do not occur separately from each other in our natural foods. So, to avoid confusion I prefer to describe the different Carbohydrate foods as either Non-Starchy or Starchy, as follows:

> **Non-Starchy** – Because these may have a significant amount of Simple Carbs they are sometimes referred to as such. But in their Fresh or Unrefined state these Simple Carbs occur in Fruits and Vegetables along with Complex Carbs, especially Insoluble Fibres and Soluble Fibres. So, they are a mix of both Simple and Complex Carbs.
>
> However, when Fresh Fruit or Vegetables contain only small amounts of Starchy Carbs or none at all we can refer to them as our Non-Starchy Carbs as shown in Table 20 on the following page.
>
> **Starchy** – Because these foods include a mix of all the Complex Carbohydrates they are sometimes referred to as such.
>
> In their Fresh or Unrefined state these foods also contain both Insoluble and Soluble Fibres in varying amounts.
>
> They may also contain small amounts of Simple Sugars, or none at all. But these foods do contain significant amounts of different Starches. So, we can refer to these as our Starchy Carbs, as shown in Table 20.

We can also consider our Non-Starchy and Starchy Carbs in terms of the amount of cooking and processing they may require to be converted to edible foods. And indeed, the extra amount of processing they may be subjected to as we humans have found new processing methods.

As we read down the column marked "Unrefined" in Table 20, we can see that many of the Non-Starchy Foods, our Fruits and Non-Starchy Vegetables can be eaten either raw or with only modest cooking preparation.

Type of Carbohydrate	1. Unrefined	2. Refined or Processed
A. Simple Or Non-Starchy	Many Fruit Our Non-Starchy Vegetables	Fruit Juices Sugar High Fructose Corn Syrup
B. Complex Or Starchy	Our Starchy Vegetables Legumes Whole Grains like Wheat, Rice, Corn Whole Grain Derivatives like Bread, Pasta	Chips/French Fries Refined Rice White Bread White Rice White Pasta

Table 20 Types of Carbohydrates

However, our Starchy Foods can rarely be eaten fresh. Many Starchy Vegetables and Legumes require some modest cooking to make them edible.

But some Grains and Pseudo Cereals may require even more processing like being ground into flour before cooking.

We can represent these foods in terms of the amount of cooking and processing they need, as shown in Table 21 on the following page.

We can also note that modest cooking or processing not only makes some inedible foods edible but may also help to retain the full array of nutrients including both the Insoluble and Soluble Fibres, plus any Vitamins, Minerals and Antioxidants.

Type of Carbohydrate	Typical Foods	Level of Processing and Cooking
Unrefined Non-Starchy Carbs	Many different Fruits Our Non-Starchy Vegetables	Most can be eaten raw. Modest cooking can enhance the nutritional value.
Unrefined Starchy Carbs	Our Starchy Vegetables Legumes and Pulses Whole Grains like Whole meal Wheat, Brown Rice, Corn on the Cob Derivatives like Whole wheat Bread and Pasta	Starchy Vegetables and Legumes need some cooking to make the starches edible. Some Grains and Pseudo Cereals may be eaten after modest cooking. Grains and Pseudo Cereals may be ground into flour and cooked as Bread, Pasta and other derivatives for maximum nutritional value.
Refined Non-Starchy Carbs	Fruit Juices Table Sugar High Fructose Corn Syrup Jams & Preserves	Highly processed foods. As well as cooking they may also require additional processing all of which can result in concentrated levels of Sugars or Starches. They lose both Insoluble and Soluble Fibres changing the way they are digested. And they lose much of their Vitamins, Minerals and Antioxidants making them less nutrient dense. The Refined Starchy-Carbs may also be combined with Fats, particularly in ready-made and packaged foods.
Refined Starchy Carbs	Refined Grains like White Flour, White or Milled Rice, Corn flour Refined Grain Derivatives like White Bread, White Pasta Many Pastries & Cakes	

Table 21 Unrefined to Refined Carbohydrates

However, as the level of processing and cooking increases towards the bottom of Table 21, then more and more of the extra nutrients may be lost, particularly micronutrients like the Vitamins, Minerals and Antioxidants.

Whilst it is unfortunate to lose any Vitamins, Minerals or Antioxidants, the loss of either or both types of Fibre can dramatically change how we digest the energy.

And please bear in mind that Tables 20 and 21 are simplified for illustrative purposes. The array of Carbohydrate foods is truly vast.

Complexity of the Carbs and the Glycaemic Index

Rather than getting in a muddle differentiating between Simple/Non-Starchy and Complex/Starchy, we can consider our Carbs in terms of the overall complexity of the foods.

At the top of Table 21, we can eat our Carbs straight off the plant after picking. Maybe we could even say "as nature intended". Although the fruits and vegetables contain the energy we need in the form of Simple Carbs, the foods also contain a mix of Insoluble and Soluble Fibres, together with nutrients like Vitamins, Minerals and Antioxidants. In other words, they have a complexity, and this complexity helps regulate how quickly and effectively we digest and absorb the energy.

As we move down the Table we come to our Unrefined Starchy Carbs. We do need to cook or process these Foods to make them edible. But if that preparation is only modest then they too retain a complexity that helps regulate how quickly and effectively we digest and absorb the energy.

However, the further down the Table we go, the more intense are the processes of cooking, refining and other preparations. As this intensity increases the foods lose more and more of their Fibres, Vitamins, Minerals and Antioxidants. These foods start to lose their complexity and as a result, the body digests them quite differently.

The Carb energy from refined Table Sugar, packaged Fruit Juices, White Bread and so on is released much more quickly into the bloodstream. This rapid release of energy is referred to as a "Sugar

Spike" and is an inefficient and unhealthy way for the body to digest and absorb the energy.

The speed with which foods may release their energy into the bloodstream may be compared using the Glycaemic Index. The Index ranks food on a scale of 1-100 indicating how quickly they release sugar into the bloodstream. Foods with a low score of 55 or less release the sugars slowly and those with a high score of 70 or more release the sugars quickly.

The absolute scores are important but must also be considered in the context of the different foods. So, determining the overall effect of the GI score can be quite nuanced.

A dedicated team at the University of Sydney in Australia maintains the official website for the Glycemic Index together with the recognized international GI database across a wide range of foods. Their website is worth a visit, **(Online Source 38).**

This is particularly important because of the impact the process has on different health conditions including Cardiovascular Disease and Type 2 Diabetes.

I must stress that I am not trying to offer any sort of dietary or health advice here. If you have any medical condition, you must consult your doctor before you make any changes to your diet.

But the impact of the different types of carbohydrate together with the effects of different levels of cooking and processing does impact on all of us. We should all strive to choose Carbohydrate Foods that release their energy in a controlled and regulated way, whenever possible.

I would suggest that it is not "Complex Carbohydrates" as such that we are looking for, but rather it is **"Carbohydrate Foods with lots of Complexity".**

How our Carbs have Changed over Time

In Chapter 24 I introduced one possible evolutionary progression for the emerging Homo Sapiens which ultimately leads to the "Modern Farmer Diet" most people eat today in one form or another.

The story started some 2.65-1.65 million years ago with the earliest Hominids who were thought to be the first "Hunter Gatherers". There is evidence they cut meat with rudimentary tools and ate a diet that also included plants, fruits and seeds.

Changes to the digestive system, mouth and teeth of the Homo Erectus some 1.9/1.8 million years ago suggest they may well have eaten cooked meat and may well have cooked roots and tubers as well.

Prof Richard Wrangham makes a compelling case for this in his fantastic book *"Catching Fire – How cooking made us human"*, **(Ref 11).**

And this ability to cook both meat proteins as well as roots and tubers for starchy carbohydrates is also inferred for the Homo heidelbergensis some 800-600 thousand years ago.

As the Homo Sapiens emerged some 300-200 thousand years ago, the evidence they ate cooked meat along with cooked roots and tubers is compelling.

It is only some 40-30 thousand years ago when the first evidence of the process of pounding grains into flour and mixing with water to produce the first bread emerges.

And it is a mere 12,000 years ago when modern agriculture emerges, and the "Modern Farmer Diet" starts to replace the "Hunter Gatherer Diet". Food like bread becomes a staple of communities and whole civilizations.

There is speculation that it was only as recently as 3,000 years BC, or 5,000 years ago that the Egyptians started to sift the flour to produce the first white flour.

And some 2,500 years ago in modern day India, where the food we now call Table Sugar was first extracted from Sugar Cane.

It is only 100 years since packaged orange juice first became widely available in the USA. And just 60 years since the introduction of High Fructose Corn Syrup as an alternative to Table Sugar.

It does seem that the evolution of the "Modern Farmer Diet" goes hand in hand with both a steady increase in the range and number of Starchy Foods in our diet together with an increase in the range and number of Refined Foods with high Sugar content as well.

Add to that the ever-expanding number of preparatory processes our Carb foods may be subjected to as well.

These changes to both our Non-Starchy and Starchy Carbs may be important factors in the evolution of the "Modern Farmer Diet" leading to one that is:

Energy rich and micronutrient poor

This evolution of our diet has brought with it some unintended consequences.

Excess Energy and rising levels of Food Intolerances

In Chapter 25 I highlighted how a number of relatively new foods may be causing a number of unintended consequences, and this is an opportune time to discuss two of these.

Eating an excessively energy dense diet – This may be one of the fundamental causes of the rising problem with obesity in this modern age and with some of the other related health problems.

It seems that as well as developing energy dense foods like grains and their derivatives, we humans just seem to go on developing the processes. Intense processes like refining grains to produce white flour strip foods of their complexity and this in turn changes the way the body processes them.

Rising levels of food intolerances and allergies – We have a growing awareness of food intolerance to some of our staple foods including:

Gluten in wheat. Gluten is a protein associated with the grains, particularly in all forms of wheat. So, the Gluten is not a Carb but is digested as a result of including grains and grain derivatives as staple foods in the "Modern Farmer Diet".

Lactose in breastmilk. Now Lactose occurs naturally in breastmilk and babies have a capacity to produce lactase, the enzyme that breaks down the lactose in the small intestine. However, babies start to lose the capacity to produce lactase as they grow.

Lactose in Dairy Foods. The introduction of Dairy Foods in some cultures introduces Lactose into the diet beyond the age when babies may stop producing Lactase. Some adults retain this capacity and can eat Dairy Foods without any issue. However, many adults do not and become Lactose intolerant.

In cultures that have included Dairy Foods over generations, the proportion of adults able to digest Lactose may be quite high. For cultures that have never included Dairy Foods, Lactose Intolerance may be almost universal.

Intolerance to some Fruits. We may be familiar with intolerances and allergies to foods like peanuts, tree nuts, gluten, dairy and shellfish. But it seems that more and more foods are joining this list. This even includes some fruit. Unfortunately for me I have developed a mild intolerance to Cherries, Peaches, and Nectarines. I have no idea what triggered it, but it is very annoying because I love Peaches and Nectarines, and my absolute favourite fruit would have to be Cherry.

It seems like we humans are building an ever-growing list of problem foods. But maybe we just need to accept that we are all different and try to work out how we can each make the most of the different food choices we now have.

Yes, we have some foods that are packed with energy, but surely the solution is to work out how to use this concentrated energy to maximum effect in our individual diets.

And just because I can't eat cherries doesn't mean my family have to stop eating them too. We can all fine tune our individual food choices whilst taking into account both food preferences and issues such as food intolerances.

Identifying Good Carbs and Bad Carbs

Although we tend to view our Carbs in terms of energy, we now know that they provide other benefits in our diet. So, trying to identify Good Carbs and Bad Carbs is not quite as straightforward as simply identifying how quickly or effectively we utilize the energy.

Good Energy Carbs

It seems that our good energy carbs are found in foods with lots of complexity. The complexity of the food allows a controlled release of energy which in turn seems to support good health.

We can find all sorts of Carb rich foods meeting these criteria. These can be Non-Starchy like Fruit and a wide range of Vegetables or Starchy like Grains, Pseudo Cereals, Legumes and some Vegetables like potatoes and yams. The important thing is to minimize any preparation and processing.

Good Carbs, our Digestive Tract and Gut Flora

Our Carbs don't just provide energy. The Insoluble Fibres and Soluble Fibres perform or rather facilitate key functions in the digestion of our food.

They help to generate Chyme with an optimal consistency allowing food to pass smoothly through the Small Intestine and which in turn allows efficient digestion and absorption of the nutrients.

Some of these Fibres also feed our good Gut Bacteria. These are our Prebiotics.

We find these fibres in our unrefined carb foods like fresh fruit and vegetables and in modestly processed grains, pseudo cereals and legumes.

Bad Energy Carbs

We find our Bad Energy Carbs in foods that have been extensively cooked and processed. These foods lose their Fibres, Vitamins, Minerals, Antioxidants and Phytochemicals. In other words, they lose their complexity, and this changes the way the body processes the energy from these foods.

Bread made from whole grain flour retains much of the complexity of the grains. But bread made with white refined flour has lost most of it. The body will utilize the energy quite differently depending on which type of bread you choose.

Bad Carbs, our Digestive Tract and Gut Flora

If our Soluble and Insoluble Fibres help generate the optimal Chyme consistency for food passing through the Small Intestine, then perhaps we can speculate what happens when the Chyme is sub-optimal.

Perhaps more worryingly though, are the High FODMAP Foods described in Chapter 19. These highly refined Carbs seem to feed or at the very least encourage the proliferation of our Bad Gut Bacteria.

This may disrupt the delicate balance that is vital to our good health. So maybe we should refer to these as our Bad Prebiotics.

It seems that we humans have developed a wide range of food choices that can provide the carbs we need for energy as well as providing Vital Nutrients for our digestive tract and gut flora. Now we can start to learn, or even re-learn, how to make the most of any and all of them.

Conflicting Effects of Modern Carbohydrates

In Chapter 23 I suggested that of all the different foods it is the Grains and particularly Rice and Wheat that symbolize the "Modern Farmer Diet". But maybe it is more accurate to say it is "The Carbohydrates".

Over the hundreds of thousands of years of evolution, our ancestors have made all sorts of inedible Carbohydrate Foods edible.

The Modern Farmer Diet came about as different cultures around the world started to cultivate key plants like Grains, Pseudo Grains and Legumes. They also domesticated animals like cattle, sheep, goats and chickens and they started to cultivate fruit and vegetables.

The rapid emergence of agriculture and the Modern Farmer Diet in all it's guises made civilizations possible.

And yet now we have taken the carbohydrates to a point where our excess processing is turning staple foods that helped build civilizations into foods that jeopardize our health.

Perhaps this is best described in terms of some of our very first carbohydrates, the Fruits.

Are Fruits really so bad for us that they make us fat?

We'll address this in the following Chapter.

30. Does Fruit really make you Fat?

I had a bizarre conversation at a local gym. The gym had a small offering of snacks and refreshments. These included various bottled drinks in a small fridge and a selection of packaged "healthy" snacks including energy bars, protein bars and flapjacks. They also had a bowl of fresh fruit.

Or rather, they used to have a bowl of fresh fruit.

But as the manager explained, he had removed the bowl of fruit because of course, "Fruit makes you fat".

I thought this was a bit extreme, but it does highlight how some messages about our diet get mixed up and become very confusing.

To get to the bottom of this we need to know how the body processes the fruit we eat and more specifically how the body processes the particular sugar most of us would associate with fruit, the Fructose.

How the Body digests Fructose

Now the Fructose in our diet may occur either as a Monosaccharide or as a constituent of the Disaccharide, Sucrose. Both may enter the small intestine, and this is where the Sucrose is broken down into its constituent parts. Now the digestion of the Fructose can begin.

> Fructose is absorbed into the bloodstream in the small intestine and is then transported to the liver.
>
> Once in the liver Fructose can be metabolized into Glucose and this Glucose can now be used for energy.

That all seems simple enough. But there is a problem with too much Fructose.

Excess Fructose in the Small Intestine

The small intestine only has a limited capacity to absorb fructose. Fructose beyond this capacity passes to the large intestine and whilst it is not toxic, large amounts of Fructose may cause uncomfortable symptoms.

Excess Fructose in the Liver

As we have already observed, fructose has to be transported to the liver where it can be metabolized into glucose.

However, the liver has only a limited capacity to process fructose. The excess fructose that can't be metabolized may be converted to fats and be laid down in the Adipose cells of our "Fat Battery". And worse still, the liver may also produce toxins if called upon to process too much fructose.

There is one more issue to take into account.

Fructose and the Calorie Deficit

Referring back to Chapter 8, we know that the body also has a limited capacity to store Glucose in the bloodstream and Glycogen in both the liver and skeletal muscle mass, which I referred to as the "Glucose Battery".

If we eat fruit when our "Glucose Battery" is already full, then this creates a problem. What happens to this excess energy?

Even if the liver has converted some of the fructose to Glucose, this extra glucose now has nowhere to go.

Well not quite, because excess glucose that cannot be stored in the "Glucose Battery" is likely to be converted to fat and stored in the "Fat Battery".

It seems that it is quite possible that we can have too much of a good thing.

It seems that fruit can be a healthy option, but we need to take some account of how we combine it with other foods and possibly even the timing of when we include it.

To understand why an apparently natural nutrient occurring in what we would consider healthy food options like fruit can possibly be a problem we need to reflect on the evolution of our species and our diet starting with the original "Hunter Gatherer Diet".

Fruits in the Hunter Gatherer Diet

We need to consider what the typical fruit intake of our distant "Hunter Gatherer" ancestors was really like.

We cannot know for sure what fruits the different tribes of Hunter Gatherers around the world were eating hundreds of thousands of years ago, or even as recently as 10s of thousands of years ago.

But we can get some idea of how much effort was involved in collecting wild fruit just from our own experiences.

Wild Blackberries

Through the summer months here in the UK, the hedgerows around the countryside will be full of wild blackberries. Now apple and blackberry pie just happens to be my absolute favourite type of fruit pie. So, the reward for picking the wild blackberries is immense.

But if you have ever done this, you will know that it takes a lot of effort to collect enough fruit just to make a couple of pies. Perhaps this is indicative of how much effort our ancestral Hunter Gatherers had to expend to collect enough fruit to make a difference to their daily diet.

Of course, you might be sceptical because the countryside here in the UK is not really that wild. So, let's consider another example.

Wild Quandongs

Whilst working in Western New South Wales in Australia, a friend had a special recipe for "Quandong Pie". The Quandong is a fruit of a particular Acacia Tree or Shrub and a favourite of the Emu. The fruit bearing Acacia looks much the same as other Acacia varieties that don't carry fruit. And because the fruit isn't brightly coloured it can be quite difficult to spot. In fact, the best way to find the fruit is to look around the base of the trees for Emu droppings. Emus love Quandongs, so lots of droppings means fruit in the tree.

Luckily, we could climb on top of the 4x4 to reach the Quandongs the Emus couldn't reach. But it still took a lot of picking to collect enough for a couple of pies. But the pies were worth it.

I appreciate that these are not universal observations and there are probably plenty of examples of fruit bearing trees and shrubs that quite naturally produce a proliferation of fruit. However, I would suggest that even when fruit does occur in proliferation, this is short lived.

If you had to "Gather" wild fruit on a regular basis, you'll more than likely need to dedicate a lot of time and effort to this activity to harvest a worthwhile amount.

Of course, this is just speculation and conjecture. But maybe we can infer from this that the human body has a limited capacity to process fructose because for most of our time on this planet we have only had limited access to foods with fructose.

So how did modern fruit come about?

Modern Fruit and Mago of Carthage

Back in Chapter 24 I pointed out that our concept of cultivated fruit is really quite recent in the grand scheme of things. Modern humans, we Homo sapiens, have been around for some 300-200 thousand years. But many of the fruit cultivation methods used to produce the big juicy fruits we know today can be traced back to the 3rd and 2nd centuries BC and the famous Mago of Carthage who is often described as "the father of agriculture".

The farming skills of the Carthaginians were a major factor in the rise of that civilization. And when the Romans defeated the Carthaginians in the Punic Wars and laid waste the city and surrounding farmland, they made sure to take the knowledge with them, preserving the works of Mago.

The Romans in turn became excellent farmers and spread this knowledge around their empire.

It seems that increasing the capacity to grow all sorts of crops including grains as well as fruits and vegetables on a large scale was instrumental in the development of civilizations.

So, what has happened, what has changed so that we reach a point where fruit may now be seen as unhealthy to eat?

Well modern fruit is not unhealthy to eat, in fact it is the complete opposite. When we eat any modern big, juicy fruit in an unrefined state, the complexity of the fresh produce, as described back in Chapter 29, should enable us to take full advantage of the nutritional content.

There may be some issues regarding what other foods we combine with fruit and there may be some issues regarding how much we eat. We'll touch on this again discussing Diet Hack 1 in a bit more detail.

But first we need to consider different ways that Fruit may now be processed and how this changes the way we digest and absorb the Fructose.

The effects of processing Fruits

We humans don't hang around. If you have anything to do with growing fruit you will know that it usually arrives all at once. And all sorts of processes have been developed to take advantage of the abundant crops of ripening fruits.

Dried Fruit

Probably the oldest and simplest method of preserving some of the fruit harvest is to dry it out.

Dried fruit can be stored to be eaten when fresh fruit is scarce or completely absent.

Most of the nutritional value may be retained in the drying process, including the Vitamins, Minerals, Fibres and Antioxidants. Indeed, the sugars help to preserve the fruit and stop it spoiling.

The one downside of dried fruit is that it produces a very concentrated food. They can have a very high calorific value by weight because the sugars are concentrated as the water is lost.

Storing Fruit in Jars and Cans

Sometimes this involves minimal preparation like peeling and slicing. Other times this may involve modest cooking such as stewing apples or pears or more involved cooking to prepare jams and chutneys for example.

That's all fine. But the preservative nature of Table Sugar means that more may be added to increase the storage life or "shelf life" to use the modern terminology.

Introduction of Packaged Fruit Juice

Packaged Orange Juice was first produced in Florida, USA, in the 1920s. What a great way to maximize the benefit of an abundant orange crop in one State and distribute it more widely.

But like the Dried Fruit, this is a concentrated food and should be treated as such.

I can recall from my own childhood that fruit juice was served in special glasses. They were smaller than regular glasses so the amount of juice served might only represent a single fruit. We enjoyed the fruit juice, but in moderation.

However, life moves on, and it became cheaper and easier to include more little luxuries like Packaged Fruit Juice. Some years back I might have served my children a modest glass of fruit juice. But left to their own devices, the children would happily serve themselves a big tumbler of fruit juice straight from the fridge. I would point out that they were drinking the equivalent of four, maybe five or even six whole fruits and that this was not healthy. I got so fed up that I stopped buying packaged fruit juice altogether.

But the fruit juices I recall from years ago was generally quite refined. The fibres and pith were removed so the juices had lost much of their complexity.

However, more recently this trend has been reversed, and many brands offer a choice of fruit juices, either "with or without the bits".

So, a packaged fruit juice that has undergone the minimum amount of processing and retained most of it's complexity, "with the bits", is healthy enough. We just need to consume it in moderate amounts.

Introduction of Reconstituted Fruit Juice

But another trend was to move on from "freshly squeezed" fruit juices to those "reconstituted from concentrates".

In other words, the original fruit juice was not only squeezed, and all the bits removed, but the bulk of the water was removed as well.

Yes, this helps preserve the concentrate and this in turn can be stored and transported more cheaply. But when the concentrate is "reconstituted" various additives are mixed in to create a product similar to a freshly squeezed fruit juice.

This end product is a long way removed from the fresh fruit we started with. It has lost most of it's complexity, probably a lot of the Vitamin, Mineral and Antioxidant content as well.

Making the Most of the Harvest and then some

Of course, one aspect of fruit growing is that the fruit ripens all at once providing a glut of produce, most of which has a very limited life. So, it is quite reasonable that we humans search for ways to use as much of the harvest as possible.

All the processes like drying, canning, preserving and juicing help us do this.

But a common theme here is that the additional processing can increase the concentration of energy whilst at the same time reduce the complexity of the foods. We can relate this back to the Glycaemic Index described in the previous Chapter. We should recognize these as concentrated energy foods and treat them with a bit of caution.

Perhaps we just need to remind ourselves that the processes we use do change the nature of the foods and how we digest and absorb the nutrients. And that some foods like "reconstituted fruit juice" may be an example of food processing going too far.

Table Sugar and High Fructose Corn Syrup

We have noted that Table Sugar is thought to have been first refined in India some 2,500 years ago. This is a highly refined food product derived from the plant we know as Sugar Cane. And it is one of the most widely traded commodities in the world.

It seems that we humans like sweet foods. In fact, we have been drawn to sweet foods for thousands and thousands of years. Different people and cultures around the world have used all sorts of sources for natural sweeteners such as:

- Tree syrups like Maple, Walnut and Birch
- Agave nectar
- Honey from Bees
- Dates

But it was the process of refining Table Sugar that brought this food to the prominence it still enjoys to this day.

Table Sugar was first refined from Sugar Cane which grows in warm climates close to the equator. An alternative crop called Sugar Beet was developed in the late 18th century and this crop could be grown in cooler climates like Europe and North America. Whilst there are some differences between the refined sugar produced from either crop, they are often both referred to as Table Sugar.

Another type of refined sugar was developed by extracting sugar from corn. The sugars were called "corn sweeteners" and were first produced in the USA in 1866. Production continued to the 1960s but was then replaced in the 1970s by another new method that produced what we now call "High Fructose Corn Syrup".

This new production method meant that the USA could produce a significant proportion of their own requirements for food sweeteners.

There may be speculation that one type of commercially produced sugar is more harmful to our health than another. But whether the sugar is derived from Sugar Cane, Sugar Beet or Corn, it is essentially the same product. All the sugars are a combination of glucose and fructose.

The issue isn't the plant source of the sweetener, it is the fact that this is a highly refined food. It has no complexity and this impacts on how the body processes it.

Sugar remains one of the most traded commodities in the world and has a long history as outlined on The Sugar Association website, **(Online Source 39)**. Rightly or wrongly people all over the world enjoy the sweetness it provides. We aren't going to change that in a hurry. But we can be aware of how we can still enjoy the benefits by treating it with caution in our own diet.

So, does fruit make you fat?

The modern concept of fruit has been a great source of highly nutritious and healthy foods that have helped civilizations grow and flourish.

However, when we start to process the fruits, we also start to lose some of those healthy benefits. And if we take these processes to an extreme like reconstituted fruit juices then we end up with a food just like refined sugar.

It may taste great, but it's not an energy source the body is designed to utilize effectively.

It seems quite reasonable to say that fruit and indeed fructose can be part of a healthy diet. But if they are processed and refined sacrificing the complexity of the original food source then, yes, they can make you fat.

But that is the same for all the carbohydrate foods.

The lesson we can all learn is to take full advantage of the wonderful foods nature and our food growers can provide for us and just be mindful to limit the degree of processing.

Now that we have covered our three macronutrients, we are ready to start pulling all this together. In Part 6 we start building our own 3 Diet Hacks and planning a diet we can live with.

And as for the risk of fruit making you fat, well when we move onto Diet Hack 1, we talk about how we can optimize the value of the fruit in our diet.

Part 6 – How 3 Diet Hacks can provide all our nutrients

31. Start Planning with 6 Food Priorities

We all need more than just Calories and Macronutrients

Starting our nutritional planning counting calories is a bit like adding fuel to a car. Yes, the car needs fuel, but it also needs different lubricants and fluids to make each of the many special functions work even before it can move, as shown in **Fig 8** below.

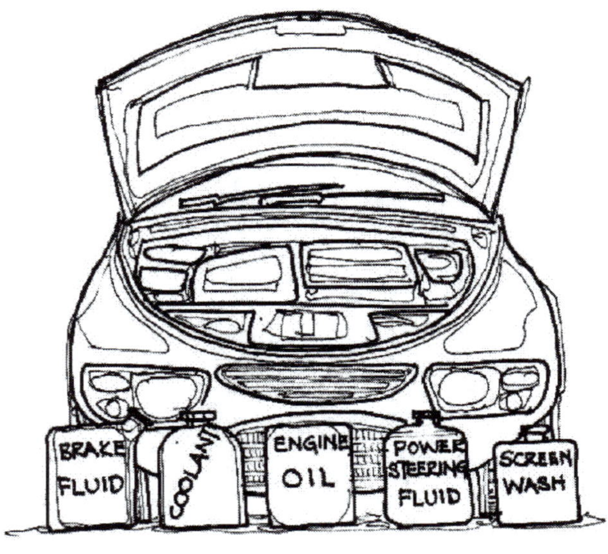

Fig 8. All the extras you need to make a car move

The human body is no different. We need a lot more than just the carbs and fats to provide energy and proteins to build our skeletal muscle.

It doesn't matter if your requirements lean towards the carbs and fats for more energy, or the proteins for more strength work, you still need

all your **"Essentials", "Non-Essentials"** and **"Vitals"**, and especially the full range of amino acids. These are the foundations of a truly balanced diet.

As we appreciate the range of the "Essential, Non-Essential and Vital Nutrients", the challenge to include them all in our regular daily food intake can seem daunting. But now we can tackle this head on, as in **Fig 9** below:

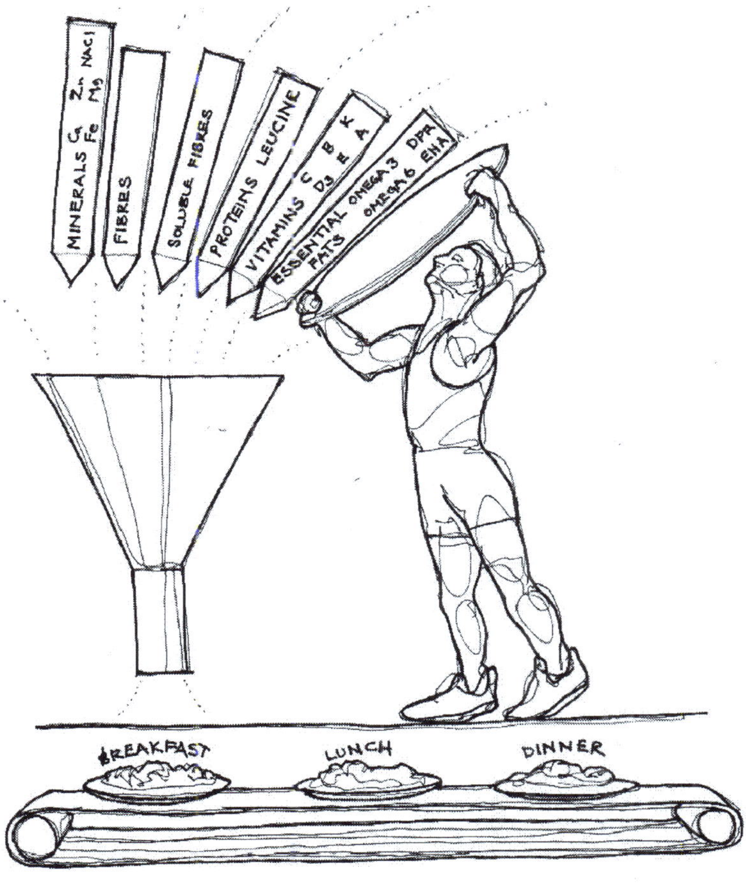

Fig 9. Including all your nutrients.

As I set about trying to include all these base nutrients, I kept asking myself if there was any particular order I should follow. I finally worked out that I was tackling this the wrong way round.

The Wrong Way Round

Right at the start of Chapter 1 I talked about taking advice from various clinical dieticians and how that advice prompted me to focus on 3 Guidelines which I listed as follows:

- Aim for 2,500 calories a day.
- Mix your Macros: Carbs 50% | Fats 35% | Proteins 15%
- Eat 5 portions of fruit & veg a day.

Starting out, the emphasis was very much on the first two:

1. Aim for 2,500 calories a day.
2. Mix your Macros: Carbs 50% | Fats 35% | Proteins 15%

I must be brutally honest and admit that the "5 a day" was a bit like an extra added on at the end and was more along the lines of "eat a variety of fruit & veg every day". As I explained in Chapter 20 the concept of "5 a day" only emerged after 1991. But because it has become such a familiar concept, I have used it throughout the book.

Now, as I struggled to recover from the tropical illness, I quickly realized I was tackling this the wrong way round. Of course, my condition was extreme, but when my small intestine wasn't working, then nothing else really worked.

When I switched my primary focus from **"calories & macronutrients"** to the **"micronutrients & vital nutrients"** everything changed. It was like finding the "on switch".

As I focused on "eating a variety of fruit & veg", my number one guideline rapidly became:

1. Eat 5 portions of fruit & veg a day.

Using this as the new starting point, I found myself looking at all my daily food in terms of my base nutrients and where I could find them in my regular diet.

I was now looking at my whole diet in a completely different way and this approach evolved into my 6 specific food priorities.

My 6 Food Priorities

Now we can explore the 6 Food Priorities and top of the list is:

1. **A selection of fresh non-starchy vegetables and fruits to provide many of my essential vitamins and minerals, most of my vital nutrients and some of my energy too.**

Many sources, including the World Health Organization (WHO), suggest a minimum of 5 portions a day of fresh vegetables and fruits. Some reputable sources suggest more. But as we covered in Chapter 20, I will be more specific and refer to 5 portions of non-starchy vegetables and fruits. as my starting point.

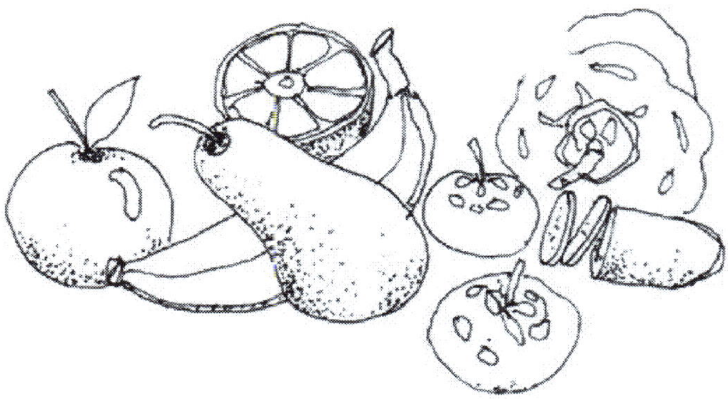

Fig 10. The stars of your diet

Most people will be familiar with the importance of these foods for our Vitamins, Minerals and possibly the Antioxidants and Phytochemicals too. But these fresh foods also contain significant amounts of both Insoluble and Soluble Fibres.

In Chapter 16 I highlighted how some Fibres perform important functions enabling the Small Intestine to work efficiently. And in Chapter 17 we covered how some Fibres feed the microbes of the Microbiome. Those preferentially feeding the good Microbes are called the Prebiotics and are important for our overall health.

It can be a challenge dealing with the logistics of larger volumes and greater variety of vegetables and fruits, be they fresh, frozen, tinned, canned, or jarred. But this is the key change you can make to your diet right now and will form the basis of Diet Hack 1.

2. A wide variety of Proteins in modest and measured portions to build and maintain my muscles and to support other key functions.

This is the one food type we can all measure out in quite careful quantities. If you eat "way too much" protein in any day, it is actually just a waste because your body can only use so much. Conversely if you eat too little or include insufficient variety then your body may struggle to maintain all sorts of key functions. However, we can all make a reasonable estimate, and you can average out your Proteins over a few days or a week, as I do.

There is a wide range of protein foods to choose from. We might typically see these as "Meat, Fish & Egg" and "Milk & Dairy" type foods illustrated in **Fig 11** below.

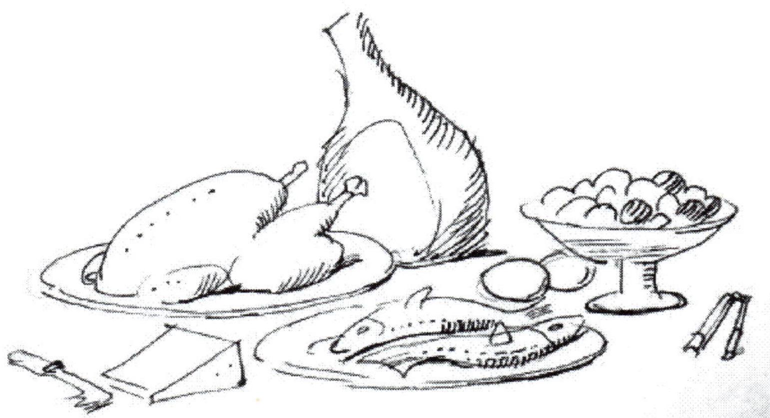

Fig 11. The Protein Foods

It is rather difficult to convey the plant-based proteins in an illustration. Even so, the range includes Seeds, Tree Nuts, Beans, other Legumes, Grains, Pseudo-Grains and concentrated foods like Tofu, Tempeh and Mycoproteins like Quorn

There are many animal-based foods with high levels of protein and many of which are "Complete Proteins". But there are only modest numbers of plant-based foods with equivalent levels. However, this doesn't detract from that huge range of plant based foods from legumes to tree nuts that can form the cornerstone of a vegetarian or vegan diet.

The total amount of protein we each need will vary depending on all sorts of criteria including gender, age, weight and activity levels. We can all make a good estimate of our requirements from a combination of the USDA guidelines and other factors which we covered back in Chapter 27 and will cover again shortly.

It is equally important that we all eat a variety of protein foods on a regular basis because **we all need the full range of amino acids.**

The proteins are so important to our health that they will form the basis of Diet Hack 2.

3. A selection of Concentrated Carbohydrates in surprisingly modest amounts to top up my key glucose/glycogen energy battery.

It might strike you as odd that I refer just to Carbs in terms of my energy. I am not ignoring the fats in my diet, it's just that I find measuring them is tricky. I will come back to them in Priority 6.

Now it doesn't matter if I am having a quiet, restful day or a physically active day I need to top up the day-to-day energy I store in my glucose energy battery. But because my "5 a Day" already includes Carbs, I'm just topping up with my Concentrated Carbs.

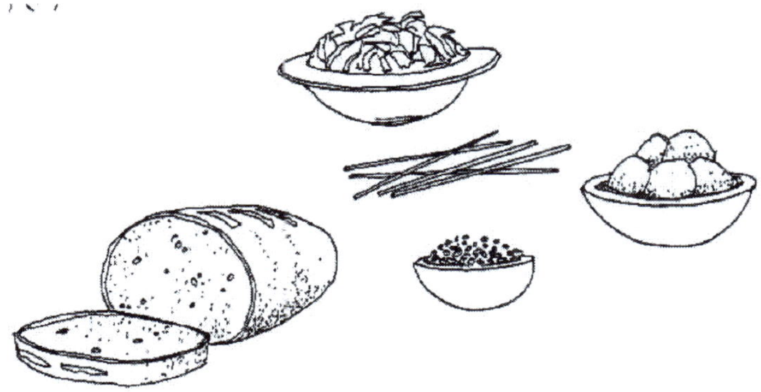

Fig 12. Bread, pasta, rice, potatoes

But look, I am not specifically talking about a "Low Carb Diet" here, I prefer to think of it more as an "Optimum Carb Diet". Carbs are an important source of day-to-day energy, but we all need to be aware of how much energy and what type of energy can be packed into some of the Concentrated Carb Foods.

There are two BIG considerations with the Carbs as described in Chapter 29 and these are:

- The amount of energy packed into many Carb Foods
- The complexity of the Carb Foods which determines how quickly the body utilises the energy.

My preference is to go for the less refined and less processed foods for my Carbs. Not only do they provide a more balanced energy source, but they are also great sources for other nutrients like fibres, vitamins and minerals. If the non-starchy vegetables and fruit provide my "5 a Day", then my Concentrated Carbs can contribute to my "6-9 a Day" suggested back in Chapter 20.

And how much Carb? We'll come back to this in Diet Hack 3.

4 Regular sources of both Vitamin D and Vitamin B12

These two Vitamins are critical for everyone, so much so that **they act as a touchstone for us all**. They highlight how **we all need to take care** to monitor all our Vitamins and all our Minerals too.

At the start of my own journey, I scanned through all the food in my regular diet to see if I was missing or low on any Vitamins or Minerals. I felt quite confident about them all except Vitamin D.

Even though we can synthesize Vitamin D in the body, some 20-30% of the UK population are deficient in this important Vitamin. I realized that I may well be in this group through the winter months, so I made sure to and still do include food sources of this Vitamin in my regular diet. Fortunately for me I like eggs and salmon and more recently have also included raw grass-fed milk.

But Vitamin D is rarely found in fruits or vegetables, apart from exceptions like blueberries and mushrooms. Fortunately, there are now fortified food options such as breakfast cereals, orange juice and coconut milk which may be especially important for vegans and vegetarians. And look, I may even take a Vitamin D supplement through the winter months.

Two close family members chose to follow a vegetarian diet and as I followed their progress, I became aware of the importance of Vitamin B12. This Vitamin has a very particular characteristic, it can only be processed by the body in small amounts. So, we must all include small amounts of Vitamin B12 in our diet every day.

This is important for everyone but may present an issue for Vegetarians and Vegans because again there are few plant-based options. However, whilst there are limited options with fresh foods there are now many "Fortified" food sources including plant-based milk substitutes like "Almond milk" and "Coconut Milk," together with fortified foods like processed "Breakfast Cereals".

For anyone following or looking to follow a vegan or strict vegetarian diet I urge you to refer back to page 46 and read the open letter published on vegan.org, **(Online Source 9).**

The spirit of the letter highlights the message for ALL of us to take care to monitor all our Vitamins and our Minerals.

5 Include sources of all the Omega 3 Fatty Acids and modest amounts of Omega 6 Fatty Acids for my brain, cells and other key functions

We only need to eat modest amounts of the different Omega 3 and Omega 6 polyunsaturated fats, but they present us with contrasting conundrums.

Many plant, seed and nut sources can provide us with the parent Omega 3 ALA, which is an essential nutrient in it's own right. But the specific Long Chain Omega 3s, EPA and DHA, present us with the first conundrum.

We have covered in some detail how EPA and DHA are essential for our brains and other key functions. The body does have the capacity to synthesise the specific Long Chain Omega 3s from the parent Omega 3 ALA, however, the process is inefficient. This means that it is unlikely that we are able to synthesize our full daily or regular requirement.

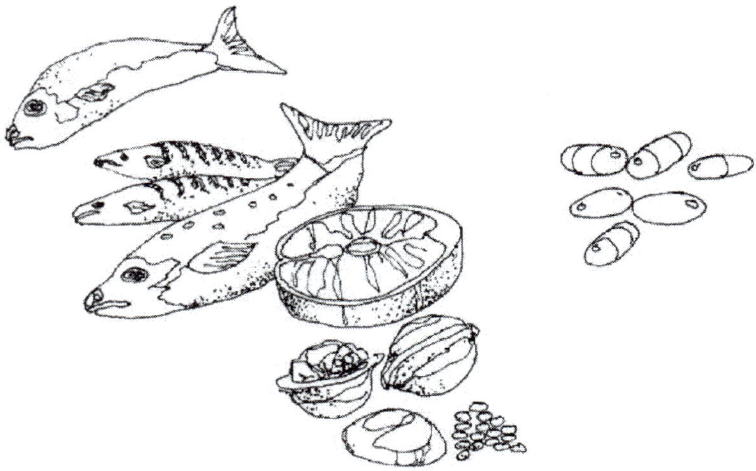

Fig 13. Fish, seafood, walnuts, seeds and capsules

Seafood and fish, on the other hand, are the best source of both EPA & DHA. Indeed, the Harvard T.H. Chan School of Public Health in the USA and the NHS in the UK both recommend that we include at least two portions of oily fish such as salmon, every week for adequate levels of EPA & DHA. For those not eating enough fish, the Harvard T.H. Chan School of Public Health even recommends regular supplements.

Interestingly research from the 1995 National Nutrition Survey in Australia shows that some "43% of their LC omega-3 PUFA was derived from red meat including beef and lamb" as reported by Peter Howe, Jon Buckley and Barbara Meyer in their paper titled "Long-chain omega-3 fatty acids in red meats" published online **(Online Source 40).** It seems that not so long ago much of the population gained nearly half of their EPA & DHA from eating meat and organ meat, particularly Beef and Lamb.

So, there are many fish and seafood sources of EPA and DHA, some meat-based sources plus fish or krill-based supplements. But there are no plant-based food sources for anyone following a vegan or vegetarian diet. There are, however, algae-based supplements that are certainly worth considering.

Omega 6 Fatty Acids also present a conundrum. The Omega 6 derivative Arachidonic Acid., AA, appears to work in tandem with DHA in the brain and with EPA in the vascular system, suggesting that it is an important nutrient in it's own right.

AA is found in different animal foods including beef, chicken, pork and eggs, sometimes occurring with EPA & DHA. Even so, meat is often ignored as a source of these essential nutrients and there seems to be unrelenting pressure to reduce the amount of meat, and especially red meat, in everyone's diet.

Only the parent Omega 6, LA, is found in plant-based foods and as with Omega 3, the process to convert the parent Omega 6 to the derivative AA is very inefficient. Furthermore, as noted in Chapter 28, including too much of the parent Omega 6 could be a problem because the optimal ratio of Omega 6 to Omega 3 should be somewhere between:

1:1 to 4:1

However, a number of recently introduced foods such as seed-based oils like rapeseed (canola) and sunflower oil have very high levels of Omega 6 relative to the Omega 3. As well as replacing animal-based products like butter, these are also used extensively in processed foods. As a result, it is now easy to get too much of this essential nutrient with some researchers now observing ratios in the order of:

16:1

There is a growing concern that such high levels of Omega 6 pose a health risk. It seems that some of the new "healthy" foods need to be treated with a little care and this leads into Food Priority 6.

6 A selection of other specific fats in modest amounts for a balanced energy supply and other key functions

We are finally seeing some sensible balance in the debate around the fats. This is very encouraging because as well as the 4 Essential Polyunsaturated Fats in Food Priority 5, we all need a variety of other fats in our diet, and we need them for a host of reasons including the following:

- Fats are important source for our energy.
- The balance between dietary fats and carbs is essential for optimal energy production for each and every one of us.
- Fats are building blocks of key hormones such as Estrogen, Testosterone and Human Growth Hormone.
- 4 of our Essential Vitamins are fat soluble.

The virtues of plant-based fats with combinations of monounsaturated and polyunsaturated fats are well documented. I am happy to include fruits like Olives and Avocados or various Tree Nuts or Legumes in my diet.

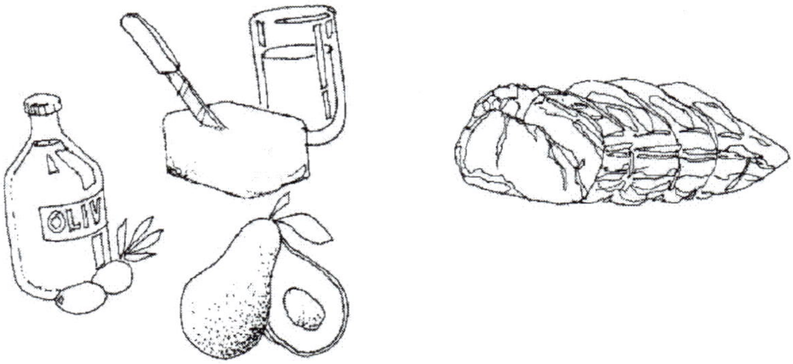

Fig 14. Olive oil, avocado, butter, milk, meat & tree nuts

But we also need some of the saturated fats and fortunately it now seems that foods such as butter are being allowed back on the table.

And let's not forget that for our average male eating 2,500 calories per day, the recommendation is that 35% should be Fats. This equates to 875 calories which in turn equates to 97 gms or 3.4 ounces. And for our average lady eating 2,000 calories per day this equates to 700 calories which in turn equates to 77 gms or 2.7 ounces of different fats.

I do personally include modest amounts of fats from meat and dairy foods. But the important caveat is that the saturated fats still need to be treated with some care.

However, by taking a little care to know what fats are in what food groups I feel confident I am including a good mix. I do take care to monitor how much of the Long Chain Saturated fats I include from any of the meats and dairy products in my diet, especially because I do want the Vitamins they host. But I am cautious about including too much of any Fats with high Omega-6 levels.

It is the man-made trans fats that need to be treated with the utmost care and avoided if possible. These generally appear in the heavily processed or "prepared foods" that fill so many shelves, fridges, and freezers in every supermarket.

One point I would stress is that I did find and still find that unlike the Proteins and the Carbs, the Fats are quite difficult to measure, especially because they are "extra" constituents of so many "prepared foods". The Food Industry has found that consumers prefer the "taste & texture" of foods with a Fat/Carb combination and the Fats, particularly the Trans Fats, can help extend "Shelf Life".

And, as well as being used in so many "prepared foods", the man-made Trans Fats are also a vital ingredient in so many pastry products. In fact, they are the very Fats that make some of the pastries so delectable, which makes for a bit of a diet dilemma.

But look, when I'm following my 3 Diet Hacks I can enjoy the occasional pastry without any feeling of guilt, so it is not the end of the world here.

Simplifying the 6 Food Priorities

My 6 Food Priorities just sort of fell into place as I explored my nutrition options. They helped me identify the range of foods I needed to build a balanced and nutritious diet.

Now I needed to bring them together into a simple framework that I could use every day, which brings us to:

Testing how I could use my 6 Food Priorities

Developing and refining my 6 Food priorities was a cathartic exercise. I found myself looking at my food in a completely different way. My daily diet was now all about selecting and combining my food intake to provide all the nutrients I needed in roughly the right amounts and proportions each day.

However, they were still a bit cumbersome to use each day and for every meal or snack.

I realised that for this to work for me, I had to keep it all as simple as possible. I needed a framework I could easily live with every day and one that helped make my food fun and enjoyable.

The framework also had to be flexible to cater for different sorts of days. There might be days when:

- I was busy but not particularly physically active.
- I was definitely going to be physically active all day.
- I just wanted to lounge around and chill.
- I was just too busy to dedicate too much time and effort to my nutrition.

As I continued testing out different approaches, I found that my Food Priorities 1 and 2 were so important that I did have to continue with these as stand-alone guidelines.

But then the Food Priorities 3-6 sort of fell together as I planned out my food, not just each day but over any given week as well.

Now this wasn't a detailed plan of every item of every Food Type in every meal and snack. No, it was more like a loose plan or roadmap based around my levels of activity.

My priorities 3-6 just seemed to get wrapped up together. Please just bear with me and it will all start to make sense as we start to explore the 3 Diet Hacks in a bit more detail.

Guidelines, Priorities and 3 Diet Hacks

When I started out, I was trying to make sense of 3 Guidelines offered by the clinical dieticians I told you about back in the Introduction. I'll refer to them again here and present them in this order:

1. Eat 5 portions of fruit & veg a day
2. Mix your Macros: Carbs 50% | Fats 35% | Proteins 15%
3. Aim for 2,500 calories a day

I found these too vague to provide a framework I could use on a daily basis. And yet the idea that I could capture the whole essence of a healthy diet in just a few clear guidelines/rules/hacks was appealing.

And now my 6 Food Priorities enabled me to do that as 3 Diet Hacks:

Diet Hack 1 - Eat a variety of fresh non-starchy veg & salad in 4 generous portions and fruit in modest portions – based on my Food Priority 1.

Diet Hack 2 - Count my proteins (and include a wide variety) – based on my Food Priority 2.

Diet Hack 3 - Plan my meals (to cover my optimum energy calories each day) – Food Priorities 3-6.

Walking you through the 3 Diet Hacks

I appreciate that we have covered a wide range of issues and topics relating to diet, some of them in considerable detail. There is a lot to take in and it might seem quite daunting.

So, over the following 3 Chapters I will walk you through how I use each of the Diet Hacks and how just about anyone can adapt them too. Hopefully you will see that I use them as three tools to build and maintain an optimum diet in line with whatever I'm up to or whatever life is throwing at me.

But this is not a chore for me. I enjoy my food, I always have. My overall aim is to include all the nutrients I need in roughly the right amounts from food I enjoy eating.

And after the trial and tribulations I went through all those years ago I appreciate the fact that by looking after my small intestine and my gut flora I can also enjoy simple pleasures like:

- A beer or two
- A glass of Rioja if it's a wine sort of day
- Sticky Toffee Pudding, with Custard of course
- Freshly picked Asparagus lightly steamed with a small knob of butter and a sprinkle of ground black pepper.

So, I can enjoy the healthy stuff and the occasional less healthy stuff, but I just don't feel like over-eating. I don't find myself craving after those "moreish foods" that fill most of the shelves in every supermarket. I can take them or leave them.

But I do find myself searching out the foods that will nourish me and satiate me. And the 3 Diet Hacks help me easily plan out meals that provide me with roughly the right amounts. They help me maintain:

A diet that provides me with elegant sufficiency

Enough of the study and preparation, now we can walk through each of the 3 Diet Hacks so you can start to build:

A diet You Can Live With.

32. Diet Hack 1

Food Priority 1 becomes Diet Hack 1

The message to include "5 a day" has become muddled. In fact, so much so that some "heavily processed foods" are even advertised as providing "one of your 5 a day". And some reputable sources include grains and legumes rightly or wrongly. But now we can be much more specific with:

> **Diet Hack 1 - Eat a variety of fresh non-starchy veg & salad in 4 generous portions and fruit in modest portions – based on my Food Priority 1.**

My baseline is to find ways to include at least 4 generous portions of non-starchy vegetables and/or salads in my daily diet and a couple of modest portions of fruit.

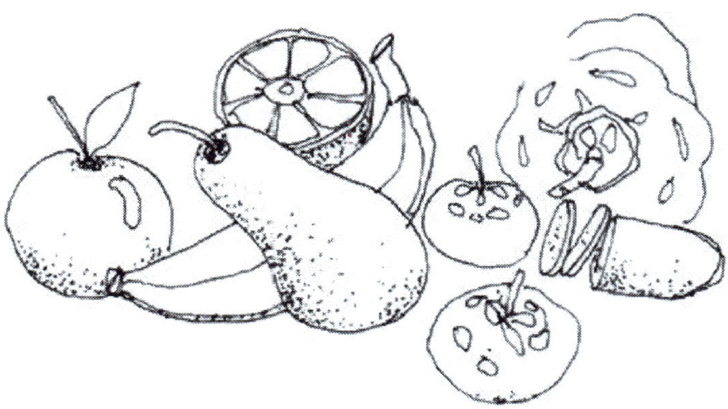

Fig 10. The stars of your diet ***(Repeat from page 205)***

Some days I don't make it, but not to worry, I'll just have a bit more the following day or over a couple of days. It's not the end of the world.

But I do understand that the thought of buying, storing and preparing enough fresh fruit and veg every day is daunting, and it is going to feel like hard work at first. So, let's start with what we mean by "fresh."

Redefining the term FRESH

In an ideal world the gold standard for FRESH vegetables and fruits would be where we can pick our chosen items freshly each day just as they reach their perfect ripeness. Of course, this is easier said than done.

But we can take advantage of the modern systems for storing and transporting fresh produce. Progress, particularly in specialized storage facilities, has enabled food outlets and supermarkets in many countries and areas to offer a much wider range of "fresh" produce throughout the year. This can even include out-of-season high value produce items being transported from across the globe. Indeed, this is a lucrative and important trade for many developing countries.

Whilst we might try to include "fresh" produce and strive for the gold standard whenever possible, it is important to remember that frozen, tinned, canned and jarred produce can be just as nutritious.

In fact, I can't stress enough that most types of frozen produce are harvested just as they reach their peak ripeness and are then processed immediately. They are literally taken from the field to the processing plant within hours. As a result, they retain a high percentage of their vitamins, minerals, antioxidants, phytochemicals and fibres.

So please bear in mind that most frozen veggies and fruit can be just as nutritious as the "fresh" produce on display, and sometimes they may even retain more micronutrients.

But it is also true that the freezing process can affect the texture. So, we just need to be creative to make the most of them. For example, frozen fruits might not work so well in terms of texture, but frozen berries are great for smoothies. I find frozen veggies are great to add to soups, broths and casseroles.

And there are many tinned, canned or jarred options too. Again, the produce is often processed immediately after harvesting so they also retain all the micronutrients and the fibres.

It is a good idea though to just check the labels to make sure there are minimal amounts of additives or preservatives like sugars, cornflower, High Fructose Corn Syrup, hydrogenated fats and of course a dreaded assortment of the E numbers.

Single Item Foods

So how can you determine the level of processing with frozen, tinned, canned or jarred foods?

I like the term "single item food". In the same way that you might examine a fresh carrot or apple, you can also examine frozen, packaged, tinned, canned or jarred foods. If you can readily see that it is for the most part a "single item food" or combination of "single item foods", and you have checked for minimal amounts of additives, then you can probably consider the item as one of your "5 a Day".

If it comes with some heavy sauce or juice or is mixed with other food items, I would be inclined to treat it as one of my "6-9 a Day".

Multi-Layered Steamer and the Wok

Much as I like a tasty salad, I generally prefer cooked veggies and am a big fan of the book *"Catching Fire"*, **(Ref 11).** And there are loads of ways to prepare the veggies too: You can boil, steam, bake, roast, sauté, stir fry even. My favourite is the multi-layered steamer in Fig 15 below.

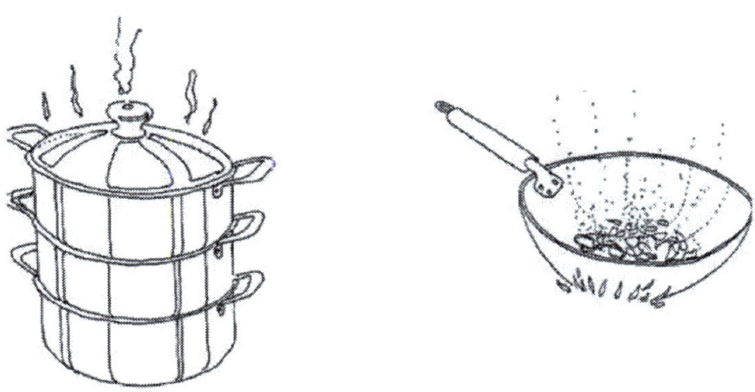

Fig 15. Multi-Layered Steamer and the Wok

I can prepare a mix of veggies using the layers to cook the different veggies for their specific ideal times. So easy and so versatile.

And it is so easy to include veggies if you are roasting. Of course, I still like my roast potatoes, but I'll also happily include other less starchy Carbs like various squashes and pumpkins and non-starchy Carbs like carrots, parsnips, beetroots, and onions and shallots too. Once you have worked out how long each needs to cook, then you just chuck them in at the right time and the end result is a great mix of veggies.

And when our kids were younger, they liked their veggies stir fried in a Wok, see Fig 15. My wife and I did have a quiet chuckle as they wolfed down stir-fried veggies including their arch nemesis cabbage.

And that reminds me that the Wok is also great for stir frying various "sprouting" foods like Alfalfa, Mustard, Cress, Watercress, Buckwheat Greens and so on.

Whilst these "sprouting" foods may not be widely available, we did find that some friends enjoyed the process of growing trays of different "sprouting" foods. And these can be great sources of Vitamins, Minerals and Antioxidants in particular.

A Pleasant Surprise

There is one very pleasant surprise in store. As you eat more "single item foods" you start to notice the variations in flavour and texture. Suddenly boring old fruit & veg becomes a real pleasure as you start to rediscover foods you had come to see as dull and boring.

I mean, one of my favourite times of year here in the UK is the "Asparagus Season". For 3 maybe 4 weeks of the year you can buy freshly picked asparagus. My absolute favourite vegetable. Lightly steamed with a smidgen of melted butter and light sprinkle of black pepper. Bliss.

How to Include 4 Generous Portions

Now you might be wondering how you can possibly include 4 generous portions of veggies in your daily diet throughout the week.

I suspect that this may be the biggest hurdle for many people, and this does require quite a shift in your expectations of your meals.

Eating out at a restaurant recently I ordered a dish with a selection of vegetables. The chef's idea of a selection of vegetables did indeed include three different vegetables. They were steamed to just the right combination of soft/crisp and tasted delicious.

However, the servings were so small the combined portion of all three would only just make up my own idea of a single "generous portion".

They were more like a dressing or garnish to the main protein and carb items on the plate. Hmm!

The shift in your expectations is to view your vegetables and salads as a substantial portion of your meal.

For my main meal of the day, I try to include the equivalent of three "generous portions", and these will fill one half of the plate, at least. And sometimes I have more because the veggies are so good.

My wife is lighter than me and less active. Her veggies also fill half the plate. But because she eats less than me, she just uses a smaller plate.

If my meals go to plan, then all I have to do is add a portion of salad into a sandwich or whatever I'm eating for a second meal. There are all sorts of items you can eat as salads, like tomato, celery, cucumber, shallots, beetroot and things like carrot sticks or grated carrot.

So Many Options

If that still sounds daunting let's just consider a few other options. For example, how many recipe books have all sorts of delicious dishes like ratatouille, or Spanish pisto, or Italian caponata? The list is endless so I'm sure you will find a few you will love. And now you know to also eat bigger portions of veggie dishes than you might have done previously.

Or you can include vegetable soups and broths in your weekly meal planning. Of course, I don't know what you have available locally, but a number of the supermarkets here in the UK carry extensive ranges of readymade soups and broths which can act as a great veggie boost as well. And, as I said before, I like to add extra frozen items to increase the veggie content.

And if you like stews and casseroles, then just add more chunky bits of cut up veggies or frozen veggies again for the final part of the cooking process.

I urge you to just start experimenting. Use Table 11 from Page 106 to help select non-starchy vegetables and fruits you want to include in your expanding range. And use Table 22 on the opposite page to jot them down.

A Note About Fruit

In Chapter 30 we covered how our digestive system has a limited capacity to process Fructose. So, what is the point of eating a wonderful piece of fruit at the end of the meal and run the risk of that perfectly nutritious Fructose ending up in your Fat Battery?

I eat my fruit when I know I can get the maximum benefit from it. That might be first thing in the morning or as a snack between meals. In fact, I find fruit a great addition to any post training snack or as a snack to nibble on if I'm out hiking for any distance.

And maybe it is just me, but I find it is very refreshing to eat fruit in this way. The juice is hydrating, and my small intestines seem to like getting the fibres that help them work efficiently. Whereas, if I ever eat fruit on a full stomach, I just find it leaves me bloated and unsatisfied.

Anyway, that's how I feel about it and I'm sticking with my fruit strategy.

When it comes to Fruit Juice, I do enjoy drinking Fruit Juice, especially freshly squeezed. But I am conscious that any Fruit Juice is an energy packed food, and it is easy to drink too much. So, I stick with the simple idea of just using a small glass that should equate to one single portion of fruit at most.

Including the "6-9"

When I get to Diet Hack 3 I am always looking for ways to include extras like legumes, beans or whole grains for my Concentrated Carbs. I see these as a chance to add to the "6-9 a Day" suggested by our friends at Oregon State University.

Plant Part	Examples	Foods I Eat	Frequency
Fruits	Sub acid - apple, stone fruit, oranges		
	Berry and Berry like – Grapes, Blueberries, strawberry, Cranberry,		
	Starchy, alkali and fatty like avocado, olive, banana, dates		
	Savoury Fruit like tomato, bell peppers, pumpkin, cucumber		
Flowers and Buds	Broccoli, Green Beans, Cauliflower, Courgettes, Sweet Peas		
Leaves	Cabbage, Kale, Spinach, Water Cress, Lettuce, Chard		
Stalks and Stems	Celery, Asparagus, Rhubarb, Kohlrabi, Leek		
Bulbs	Onions, Shallots, Garlic,		
Roots and Tubers	Beets, Carrots, Turnips, Sweet Potatoes, Yams, Parsnip		
Fungi	Mushrooms, truffles,		

Table 22 Your Salads, Fruits, Non-Starchy Vegetables

And some days I find I've included all my "5 a Day" plus some of my "6 9". But other days I don't quite make it. Since I feel so much better for making it, that's a huge incentive for me to strive for that each day.

Enjoy the Journey

And do remember that things are never simple.

For example, some Roots and Tubers may be better classified as Starchy Veggies or may sit somewhere between Starchy and Non-Starchy. Some legumes like the pea may be referred to as veggies and some fruits like tomato, zucchini and melons may be referred to as veggies or salads too.

And it's the same with fruits as we touched on back in Chapter 22.

Look, the boundaries are fuzzy. This is half the fun. Just take the opportunity to explore your food options.

If I can, I like to buy fruit and veg that is "in season". But the modern transport and storage facilities have extended these seasons for different produce meaning many of us have wider choices for extended periods. And frozen, tinned and jarred veggies and fruit can be just as nutritious.

And as for portion sizes, just experiment to find what works best for you. I probably eat more than 4 portions of veggies regularly just because I enjoy them. But you might find smaller portion sizes or spreading them more evenly over two meals may work better for you.

Or you may prefer to combine them into other dishes like casseroles, ratatouille, or pisto. You probably have recipe books already that have all sorts of similar types of recipes.

There is a whole world of food to go and explore.

Who would have thought it?

The adventure of Fruit & Veg begins!

33. Diet Hack 2

Food Priority 2 becomes Diet Hack 2

Trying to measure out all your Macronutrients has a certain appeal. But they perform different functions. Whilst our energy requirements can fluctuate significantly day to day this is not the case for our genuine protein requirements which only vary modestly. We refer to this as the Calorie Conundrum discussed back in Chapter 26.

We have also covered the importance of meeting our genuine protein requirement, our **"RDA of Reference Proteins",** at some length.

This is our baseline, the minimum amount we all need to digest and absorb in order to maintain our skeletal muscle mass and a host of other important bodily functions. Getting enough protein, and all the Amino Acids, is as important as getting all our vitamins and minerals.

Furthermore, we can all make a pretty good estimate of our genuine daily requirements. And we can average this out over a few days or a week, so measuring our daily intake can be quite straightforward, whatever your food preferences. This leads to:

> **Diet Hack 2 - Count my proteins (and include a wide variety) – based on my <u>Food Priority 2</u>.**

I appreciate that "Counting Proteins" can seem daunting at first, in much the same way that "5 a Day" was too. But once you have tried it a few times it quickly becomes second nature.

Start by Estimating your Genuine Protein Requirements

My ideal weight is 160 lbs and my daily activity level ranges from leisurely to Physically Active. So, from Table 16, shown again over the page, my RDA of Reference Proteins ranges from 56 g to 82.4 g.

You can use Table 16 to estimate your genuine "RDA of Reference Proteins" based on your gender, activity level and bodyweight.

Protein Requirement for Female aged 40			
Bodyweight in lbs. ***in kgs***	**1** USDA Min requirement 0.33 g/lb. 0.72 g/kg	**2** Physically active requirement 0.51 g/lb. 1.12 g/kg	**3** Top level sport requirement 0.68 g/lb. 1.5 g/kg
100lbs ***45.5kg***	**33 g**	**50.5 g**	**68 g**
120lbs ***54.5kg***	**39.6 g**	**60.6 g**	**81.6 g**
140lbs ***63.6kg***	**46.2 g**	**70.7 g**	**95.2 g**
160lbs ***72.7kg***	**52.8 g**	**80.8 g**	**108.8 g**
180lbs ***81.8kg***	**59.4 g**	**90.9 g**	**122.4 g**
200lbs **90.6kg**	**66 g**	**101 g**	**136 g**
Protein Requirement for Male aged 40			
Bodyweight in lbs. ***in kgs***	USDA Min requirement 0.35 g/lb. 0.77 g/kg	Physically active requirement 0.52 g/lb. 1.13 g/kg	Top level sport requirement 0.68 g/lb. 1.5 g/kg
140lbs ***63.6kg***	**49 g**	**72.1 g**	**95.2 g**
160lbs ***72.7kg***	**56 g**	**82.4 g**	**108.8 g**
180lbs ***81.8kg***	**63 g**	**92.7 g**	**122.4 g**
200lbs ***90.9kg***	**70 g**	**110 g**	**136 g**
220lbs **100kg**	**77 g**	**113.3 g**	**149.6 g**
240lbs ***109.1kg***	**84 g**	**123.6 g**	**163.2 g**

Table 16. (Repeat) Activity and Protein Requirement Chart

This is a repeat of Table 16 from page 140.

And do use your "ideal" bodyweight. If you are a few pounds overweight, then take that into account. That excess weight does not need extra protein. Or add a bit if you are genuinely underweight.

Averaging My Protein Requirements over a Week

In Chapter 26 I used a typical week to show how my daily calories might vary from 2500 to 3200 depending on my physical activity levels. I then calculated my daily protein requirement. Over a week, this gave me a daily average of 74.8g, as shown in Table 17 again below.

Day	Activity	Activity Level	Daily Protein
Monday	Work + Strength w/o	Physically Active	82.4 g
Tuesday	Work + General Stuff	Average	56 g
Wednesday	Work + Strength w/o	Physically Active	82.4 g
Thursday	Work + General Stuff	Average	56 g
Friday	Work + Strength w/o	Physically Active	82.4 g
Saturday	Big Run + Family Stuff	Physically Active	82.4 g
Sunday	Recovery Run + Fam Stuff	Physically Active	82.4 g
Daily Average over the Week			**74.8 g**

Table 17. (Repeat) Estimated Activity Levels and Daily Protein

I found that averaging my proteins over a week worked for me, but just experiment to find the timeframe that works best for you.

Accounting for the Biological Value of Protein Foods

We know from Chapter 27 that we do not digest all of the proteins in our food. But we can use the measure termed the Biological Value, or BV, to determine how much protein we might expect to fully digest and absorb from any particular food as illustrated in Table 18 shown again in the following page.

Protein Food	Typical Portion	Gram of Protein /typical portion	Estimated Biological Value %	Gram of Protein actually absorbed
Whey Protein	30g scoop	20g	98	**19.6g**
Eggs	2 med size	12g	93.7	**11.2g**
Buckwheat	60g ½ cup	11.5g	90	**10.4g**
Milk	240g glass	8g	84.5	**6.8g**
Yoghurt	125g 1 cup	13g	84	**10.9g**
Cheese	2 oz/56.7g	14g	84	**11.8g**
Quinoa	85g ½ cup	11g	83	**9.1g**
Whole Grain Rice	82g ½ cup	3.3g	83	**2.7g**
Fish, salmon	3 oz/85.05g	23g	76	**17.5g**
Seafood, crab	3 oz/85.05g	17g	76	**12.9g**
Beef, rump steak	3 oz/85.05g	26g	74.3	**19.3g**
Chicken, breast	3 oz/85.05g	25g	74	**18.5g**
Tofu firm	3 oz/85.05g	14.5g	74	**10.7g**
Soya Beans, boiled	85g ½ cup	15g	72.8	**10.9g**
Mushrooms	3 oz/85.05g	3g	70	**2.1g**
Quorn	100g	12g	70	**8.4g**
Seeds, sunflower	36g ¼ cup	8g	70	**5.6g**
Legumes, chickpeas	82g ½ cup	8g	68	**5.4g**
Breakfast Cereals	28g 1 cup	2g	*Est (65)	**(1.3g)**
Whole Grain Bread	92g 2 slices	8g	64	**5.1g**
Tree Nuts, pecan	36g ¼ cup	5g	60	**3g**
Beans, dry	85g ½ cup	8g	58	**4.6g**
Lentils	90g half cup	9g	45	**4g**

Table 18. (Repeat) The Biological Value of Protein foods

Protein Food	Typical Portion	Gram of Protein /typical portion	Estimated Biological Value %	Gram of Protein actually absorbed

Table 23. The Biological Value of your Protein foods

Before we cover how to allow for the BV of the protein foods, I suggest that you use Table 18 to identify the different Protein Foods you are already including in your diet, and those you might like to include. Jot these down on Table 23 together with their Biological Values.

Now you have started to build a list of your main Protein Foods for future reference.

The easiest way to illustrate how we take into account the BV of our protein foods is to use a typical example of one of my own meal plans.

Bringing it altogether

Table 24, opposite, provides the breakdown of my own meals and snacks for a typical day. This includes the protein foods I am including and the portion sizes in the various meals throughout the day.

Then it shows the actual Protein Content of the portions, followed by the Biological Values of each food. Now I can make a good estimate of how much protein I will actually digest and absorb.

And I end up with two Protein Totals:

1. The Total Protein Content
2. The Total Absorbed Proteins

It is this second figure that I am really interested in. I can quickly determine how close I am to my average "RDA of Reference Proteins" which is shown in the second last row of the Table.

And as you can see, the meal plan for this day would leave me a little over my average "RDA". But as I average my proteins over the week, there will be other days when I may be a little under.

Or I could reduce the portion size in one of the meals or snacks.

The bottom line of the Table is interesting. "The Average BV of Total Daily Proteins" isn't an official or scientific term, but I have found this figure useful because it gives me an overview of how much of all of the proteins I am likely to absorb and digest.

	My Proteins	1. Total Protein content	BV (%)	2. Total Absorbed Proteins	Veg, Salad & Fruit
Morning Starter					Small portion of fruit Satsuma
Breakfast	2 Med eggs 2 slice of whole grain toast Greek style Yoghurt	12g 8g 13g	93.7 64 84	11.2g 5.1g 10.9g	
Lunch	1 oz grilled chicken breast 2 slices of whole grain bread Sprinkle of seeds	8.2g 8g 2g	74 64 70	6.1g 5.1g 1.4g	Stuff the sandwich with loads of salad
Post Exercise Snack	Glass of milk Handful of Cashew & Brazil nuts	8g 5g	84.5 60	6.8g 3g	Eat a Banana a little later
Dinner or Evening Meal	4 oz fish/meat ¼ cup Quinoa	34.6g 5.5g	74.3 83	25.7g 4.7g	My ½ plate of non-starchy veggies Or Plate of salad
Total Proteins		**104.3g**		**80.0g**	
My Average RDA of Reference Proteins				**74.8g**	
Average Biological Value of Total Daily Proteins		**80/104.3**	**=**	**77%**	

Table 24. Calculating My Daily Protein Intake

You can see that the amount of protein I am likely to digest and absorb is less than the total in all the foods included for the day. But we now know that is because the body cannot utilize all the proteins in our food. This is quite normal, and it is important to take this into account to make sure you do include sufficient Protein in your regular diet.

Surprisingly Modest Portion Sizes

For those of you including foods from our "Meat, Fish & Eggs" and "Milk & Dairy" Food Groups, I think you will find it quite easy to identify and measure out your main Protein Foods.

Even after taking into account that you might only digest 70-80% of the proteins in your food, you might be surprised by the portion sizes you do need to meet your RDA of Reference Proteins. Indeed, you may well find that you can now include more modest portions than you are used to up to now.

But at the same time, using the steps outlined you can be confident that you are still including something close to your optimal level of Proteins, in line with your age, gender, physique and activity level.

Furthermore, the mix of "complete proteins" and extras like the "Sprinkle of Seeds" and "Handful of Nuts" means you should be covering all your Amino Acids.

And given that these foods tend to be quite expensive, you can now focus more on the quality and sourcing.

Sample Meal Plan for a Vegetarian

Table 25 on the opposite page provides a breakdown of Sue's meal plan for a typical day. Now Sue does include modest portions of foods from the "Milk & Dairy" Group, plus Eggs. I realise that other vegetarians might prefer not to include Eggs, but just bear with me for a moment.

Discussing her meal plan revealed two things. Sue tends to:

1. Underestimate how much Protein she needs in her diet
2. Overestimate how much Protein she absorbs and digests.

	Sue's Proteins	1. Total Protein content	BV (%)	2. Total Absorbed Proteins	Veg, Salad & Fruit
Morning Starter					
Breakfast	1/3 cup Greek Style Yoghurt Corn Flakes	4.3g 2g	84 (65)	3.6g 1.3g	
Lunch	Egg Mayo Sandwich Filling 2 slices of whole grain bread Sprinkle of seeds	3g 8g 2g	93.7 64 70	2.8g 5.1g 1.4g	
Light Snack					
Dinner or Evening Meal	3 oz Tofu ¼ cup Legumes Handful of nuts	14.5g 4g 5g	74 68 60	10.7g 2.7g 3g	
Total Proteins		**42.8g**		**30.6g**	
Sue's Average RDA of Reference Proteins				**39.6g**	
Average Biological Value of Total Daily Proteins		**30.6/42.8**	**=**	**71.4%**	

Table 25. Calculating Sue's Daily Protein Intake

I was puzzled. But there seems to be a persistent message in the media making what may or may not be a reasonable generalization to suggest that people who do include "Meat, Fish & Eggs" plus "Milk & Dairy" Foods "may" have a tendency to eat more protein than they need. And that this "may" be harmful to their health.

Then conversely, we do need to consider if this is having the reverse effect for those moving away from animal-based proteins. Can the concern to avoid eating too much protein result in eating too little and any potentially harmful effects that might cause?

I was struck by how Sue, which is not her real name by the way, was very anxious to "not eat too much protein". And this is demonstrated by her meal plan in which she is only including some 30.6 g of her daily estimate of 39.6 g. This equates to just 76% of her average "RDA of Reference Proteins".

When I was discussing this aspect of diet with a wider group of vegetarians, it did seem that there was a general, albeit anecdotal, tendency to underestimate their proteins, namely by:

- Erring on the low side when estimating their RDA of Reference Proteins
- Not taking sufficient account of the lower BVs for many plant-based foods, such as Legumes, Grains or Tree Nuts
- Not measuring out the protein elements of vegetarian dishes

On the first point I would just reiterate that Column 1 in Table 16 is a minimum recommendation for people just going about their lives. It is better to include a little bit more than you need rather than run the risk of not including either sufficient protein as a total amount or not covering all your Amino Acids.

On the second and third points perhaps, we should consider this from the perspective of those following a stricter vegetarian or vegan diet. And particularly how to include "complete proteins" in their diet.

BVs and Complete Proteins for Vegetarians and Vegans

Referring back to Table 18 on page 216, we can see that many plant-based proteins may have both lower protein levels and lower Biological

Values. But we know that this is because there are fewer plant-based protein foods providing “complete proteins”.

But we don’t have to treat this as a problem, it’s more the case that we just need a different solution.

And fortunately, there are numerous reputable sites and authors showing you how to combine plant-based foods to provide more “Complete Protein” combinations. Anyone following or looking to follow a strict vegetarian diet, or a vegan diet can search out a reputable site or sites that appeal to them.

Why can’t I cover this in more detail here? There are so many choices of Grains, Pseudo Grains, Legumes, Nuts, Tree Nuts, Seeds, Mushrooms and so on that you can use as your protein source. And that means there are any number of combinations you can use to achieve “complete proteins” in your meals or throughout the day too.

The topic is huge, so, rather than me trying to muddle through, the best solution is to encourage you to find an author or site that appeals to you.

And if you are really stuck then you can always start with the Vegan Society Website, **(Online Source 9).**

Of course, using the BV Charts and Meal Planner will be less reliable because you don’t know how much the combining of different foods will increase the overall BV.

But you can always use the “The Average BV of Total Daily Proteins” from Tables 24 & 25 as a guideline, so somewhere between:

71 – 77 %

And look, this is rather like Diet Hack 1, you can treat this as a journey of exploration. Go and check out all the great food options out there.

How Vegetarians and Vegans can Get All Their Amino Acids

It is a bit like the “restaurant scenario” I described in Diet Hack 1, where the veggies were treated as a garnish resulting in smaller portions. Key Protein Foods in a vegetarian or vegan dish, such as Legumes, Grains, Seeds or Tree Nuts, are not a garnish either. You need plenty of them either individually or combined.

I would strongly suggest that you do make the effort to measure how much of any protein element you include in portions of say a "nut roast" or a "legume casserole". So do measure the individual protein items like the kidney beans, or the chickpeas, or the peas.

So, while I do understand that it is a bit more difficult to measure these out in your regular diet, it is still important to do so.

And just like my own meal plan back in Table 24, look for ways to add small helpings of Tree Nuts or Seeds through your day. This is a great way to not only meet your daily requirement as a total, but also to include a wide variety of foods to cover all your Amino Acids too.

Final Thoughts

Now I do find there is quite a lot of pressure for people to reduce their protein intake without offering any guidance on either minimum or optimum amounts.

I would, therefore, like to reiterate that the USDA Guidelines figures shown in Column 1 of Table 16 are minimum figures for absorbed Proteins for people just going about their lives.

Furthermore, when we think about our proteins, we should really think of these in terms of the full range of 20 Amino Acids we all need.

And we must remember not just the role they play building and maintaining our skeletal muscle mass, but the roles they play in the thousands of proteins throughout the body right down to each and every cell.

It is just as important to get all our Amino Acids as it is to get all our Vitamins and Minerals.

If in doubt, you can always include a little bit more. It would seem from Chapter 27 that you would have to eat a lot more than the amounts suggested here, even for the elite athletes, before there is any apparent health risk.

But eating too little on a regular basis may well have health ramifications.

And one final point. Proteins are often the focus or centrepiece of a meal and often the most expensive food items as well. So, let's make the absolute most of all the fantastic Protein Foods.

Charts for You to Use

You might find it useful to use the blank charts shown below and over the page to help with your own planning.

.

Day	Activity	Activity Level	Daily Protein
Monday			g
Tuesday			g
Wednesday			g
Thursday			g
Friday			g
Saturday			g
Sunday			g
Daily Average over			g

Table 26 Estimating Activity Levels and Daily Protein

	My Proteins	1. Total Protein content	BV (%)	2. Total Absorbed Proteins	Veg, Salad & Fruit
Morning Starter					
Breakfast					
Lunch					
Post Exercise Snack					
Dinner or Evening Meal					
Total Proteins		g		g	
My Average RDA of Reference Proteins				g	
Average Biological Value of Total Daily Proteins				= %	

Table 27 Calculating My Daily Protein Intake

34. Diet Hack 3

Food Priorities 3-6 become Diet Hack 3

Well, I already know how much fruit and non-starchy veg I'm going to eat. It's just a matter of choosing the best options. And I know what protein foods I'm going to eat and roughly how much.

All I need to do now is juggle these into meals at the best or most convenient time of day and "maybe" top up the meals with my Concentrated Carbs or include some extra Fats for my daily energy.

This simple planning process then lets me scan my overall diet to make sure I am covering all my remaining Food Priorities from 3 – 6. In other words, making sure that I have covered all my Vitamins, Minerals and Vitals. I take particular care to keep tabs on crucial nutrients like my essential Omega 6 and Omega 3s, especially DHA & EPA, as well Vitamin B12, Vitamin D, and so on. Which all leads to:

> **Diet Hack 3 - Plan my meals (to cover my optimum energy calories each day) – <u>Food Priorities 3-6</u>.**

We do need to clarify something before we start though.

Food Priority 6, a selection of Fats for Energy

We start with our Fats specifically because there seems to be pressure from so many sources pushing us to "Eat less Fat", or "Eat a Low-Fat Diet" or to even "Eat a No Fat Diet".

But there is an aspect of our fats that I need to highlight again. Our two energy foods, the Carbs and Fats, do not act in isolation.

Yes we do effectively have two different energy storage systems as we covered in Chapter 8, but the body does in fact use both carbs and fats for energy even at low levels of activity. Furthermore, reducing or cutting fats out of this equation is detrimental.

Indeed, we each have a sort of "optimal ratio" of the two that works most effectively.

And this helps explain why we are advised that something like 35% of our daily calorie intake should be made up of fats.

This equates to:

- 97 gms or 3.4 ounces for our average male eating 2,500 calories
- 77 gms or 2.7 ounces for our average lady eating 2,000 calories

However, unlike our Proteins or Carbs we don't really have any "Fat Foods" that we can measure out in the same way as, for example we might select a slice of cheese, a couple of eggs or a portion of potato.

It seems that our fats are included within certain foods and we are trying to take the various fats into account as we select portions of our different protein or carb foods and even fruits.

And of course, the cooking medium for many foods and dishes may well be one fat or another, be they from animal sources like butter and lard, or plant sources such as olive or canola oil.

So whilst we do need to take some care with our fats, we still need 2, 3, or more ounces a day depending on our gender, size and activity level. I will come back to the Fats again shortly.

Food Priority 3 – Concentrated Carbs

Back in Chapter 23, I organized the different Food Groups into 4 Categories. The high energy Starchy Veggies are paired with the high energy Grains and their Derivatives in Category 3 as shown in Table 10 which is repeated on the page opposite.

I refer to Category 3 as my "Concentrated Carbs" because that is easier to use than "High Energy + Some Protein". These are the high energy foods that I now include in only modest portions. But don't forget even these small portions still pack a lot of calories!

Category Type	Description	Origin	Food Groups
1. High Protein	These are foods with the highest levels of Protein	Animal	- Meat, Fish & Egg
		Plant	- Concentrated Plant Protein
2. Protein +Energy	Foods with relatively high Protein but similar or higher levels of energy, often derived from Fats or Oils as well as Carbs.	Animal	-Milk & Dairy
		Plant	-Tree Nuts & Seeds -Legumes & Pseudo-cereals
3. High Energy + some Protein	Foods with high Energy levels, typically from Starchy Carbs. They may contain modest to low levels of Proteins.	Plant	-Grains & Derivatives -Starchy Vegetables
4. High Vitals +some Energy	Foods with high levels of different Vital Nutrients and energy mainly as simple Carbs	Plant	-Fruits -Non-Starchy Vegetables & Salads

Table 10 (Again). Four Categories of the Food Groups

(I refer to Category 3 as my Concentrated Carb Foods)

As I re-organized my food using the 3 Diet Hacks, I was genuinely surprised how little of the Concentrated Carbs I really needed.

By covering all my "5 a Day" and my "Proteins" I found and still find that I don't need to add much by way of Concentrated Carbs for energy. The combination of Proteins and associated Fats together with all the Fibres provided by Diet Hacks 1 & 2 is very satiating and the combination provides a surprising amount of "**Carb energy"** as well.

I find myself just topping up my energy with modest portions of Concentrated Carbs in line with how active I am. And I do mean modest, as illustrated with my Food Plate at the end of this Chapter.

Whenever possible I try to select **"Carbohydrate Foods with lots of Complexity".** In other words, the "Unrefined Starchy Carbs" from the top half of Table 21, shown again on the opposite page.

So even when I add my new modest portions of Concentrated Carbs like rice, potato, pasta, beans, bread and so on, I hardly ever feel hungry between meals. And I certainly don't get cravings to eat a pile of doughnuts or chocolate biscuits or a couple of big slices of cheesecake.

And even if I should succumb to the temptation for some of those "moreish foods" that are so bad for us, well it's not a problem because:

- I will still only be able to eat a modest amount because I'm already rather full and satiated.
- Or at the worst, my digestive system will deal with them very efficiently anyway because it's been primed with Fibres, Prebiotics, Antioxidants and Phytochemicals.

This is a huge relief because I am very partial to Sticky Toffee Pudding, with Custard obviously, Crème Anglaise if you are a bit posh, and other similarly delicious puddings. And Cheesecake. And I do enjoy a beer or two on occasion or a glass of wine relaxing in the evening.

But somehow or other I just seem to have found a balance whereby I can enjoy these without needing to overindulge.

Food Priority 4 – Covering all the Vitamins and Minerals

In Chapter 11 I highlighted how Vitamin B12 and Vitamin D are really touchstones for us all. I can't recommend the open letter by Stephen Walsh of the Vegan Society highly enough. It is titled "What Every

Type of Carbohydrate	Typical Foods	Level of Processing and Cooking
Unrefined Non-Starchy Carbs	Many different Fruits Our Non-Starchy Vegetables	Most can be eaten raw. Modest cooking can enhance the nutritional value.
Unrefined Starchy Carbs	Our Starchy Vegetables Legumes and Pulses Whole Grains like Whole meal Wheat, Brown Rice, Corn on the Cob Derivatives like Whole wheat Bread and Pasta	Starchy Vegetables and Legumes need some cooking to make the starches edible. Some Grains and Pseudo Cereals may be eaten after modest cooking. Grains and Pseudo Cereals may be ground into flour and cooked as Bread, Pasta and other derivatives for maximum nutritional value.
Refined Non-Starchy Carbs	Fruit Juices Table Sugar High Fructose Corn Syrup Jams & Preserves	Highly processed foods. As well as cooking they may also require additional processing all of which can result in concentrated levels of Sugars or Starches. They lose both Insoluble and Soluble Fibres changing the way they are digested. And they lose much of their Vitamins, Minerals and Antioxidants making them less nutrient dense. The Refined Starchy-Carbs may also be combined with Fats, particularly in ready-made and packaged foods.
Refined Starchy Carbs	Refined Grains like White Flour, White or Milled Rice, Cornflour Refined Grain Derivatives like White Bread, White Pasta Many Pastries & Cakes	

Table 21 Unrefined to Refined Carbohydrates

This is a repeat of Table 21 on page 170.

Vegan Should Know About Vitamin B12" and is published on the Vegan Society website, **(Online Source 9**).

The letter carries an important message for all of us because regardless of our individual food preferences we must all seek out ways to include all our nutrients in our individual diets.

And again, we have a bit of an issue depending on our food preferences.

If you do eat foods including "Meat, Fish & Eggs" and/or "Milk & Dairy" then you have plenty of sources of both Vitamin B12 and Vitamin D.

But Vitamin D also highlights the possible downside of "Low Fat" or "No Fat" diets because it is a Fat-Soluble Vitamin. If the milk is treated to produce semi-skimmed or skimmed milk, then the fat is removed along with Vitamin D. Another example of how food processing can be detrimental to the nutritional value of our foods.

And whilst I might sometimes seem a little critical of food manufacturers, I do try to acknowledge when they do good work too.

That is certainly the case when it comes to "Fortifying" foods with both Vitamin B12 and Vitamin D as well as some of the harder to get nutrients, including Vitamin A.

Now I generally feel that with such a wide range of foods in my diet including vegetables, fruits and salads, a wide range of my preferred protein foods, together with a variety of grains and legumes, I am covering all my mineral requirements.

But it is still reassuring to know that if needs be, I can include fortified foods to also cover the harder to get minerals like Iodine and Zinc. Iron is another mineral included in fortified foods. Iron can be a problem for vegetarians and vegans, but it is another mineral included in fortified foods.

The important message here is that **we all need to take care** to cover all our vitamins and minerals. Great online sources include the Micronutrient Information Centre at Oregon State University, **(Online Source 11**) and I have my go-to copy of Jane Higdon's book, **(Ref 6).**

Food Priority 5 – the Essential Fatty Acids

Back in Chapter 10 we covered the importance of EPA and DHA. These two Long Chain Fatty Acid Omega 3s are so fundamental to the development and health of the human brain and vascular system yet they often seem to be overlooked in the modern farmer diet.

They are so important that the NHS in the UK, and Harvard T.H. Chan School of Public Health in the US both highlight seafoods and recommend at least two portions of oily fish each week. They even advise using supplements if there is not enough oily fish in the diet.

I also find it intriguing that the organ meats of "grass fed" cattle and sheep, in other words livestock grazing in their natural habitat, can also provide a significant portion of these nutrients. And yet these nutrients may be almost absent when livestock is managed by modern methods. How strange is it that "modern" livestock farming methods can have a detrimental effect on the nutritional value of the food we eat?

I have taken on board the message from *'The Chance to Survive'* discussed back on page 49, **(Ref 5),** and I have taken a leaf out of the research from Australia regarding genuine "grass fed" meats covered in page 210, **(Online Source 40).** I now try to purchase "grass fed" meat and dairy products if I can here in the UK.

I try to include oily fish, especially salmon, in my regular diet. But if I feel my diet might still be low on the key nutrients, DHA and EPA, then I may include a supplement for some months of the year.

But of course, I appreciate that this is an important issue for vegans and vegetarians because there are no plant-based options for the Omega 3 derivatives DHA and EPA. This does present a dilemma, however, there are options for supplements based on the algae that the fish and krill feed on.

There is debate around the classification of algae. Some classify algae as a type of plant, but others assign them to a group called "protists". Once again, we find the issues around nutrition are full of nuances and given that a couple of family members follow vegetarian diets, this is an issue we follow closely.

There is also confusion because some Food Adverts actively promote foods high in Omega 3 but fail to specify if they mean the parent ALA, or the two key derivatives EPA and DHA. This is an important detail because as we know from Chapter 10, the body has only a limited capacity to convert the parent Omega 3, ALA, as reported by our friends at Oregon State University, **(Online Source 5).**

There is also some confusion regarding Omega 6. It seems that the derivative Arachidonic Acid, AA or sometimes ARA, is important for both the brain and the vascular system and yet only the parent Omega 6 Linoleic Acid, LA, is considered an essential nutrient.

AA is readily available in animal-based foods like beef, chicken, eggs and pork but the parent Omega 6, LA, is only found in plants, especially in seeds. Seeds such as canola or sunflower may be used to make vegetable oils which may be used extensively in processed foods.

If you use a lot of seed-based oils or consume a lot of processed foods, you do need to be aware of the issue raised in Chapter 28 and treat these with a bit of caution.

Food Priority 6 – a selection of Fats for Energy

And as for my Fats for energy, well it's the same story as my Carbs. Because I have covered my "5 a Day" and my Proteins I can be selective about my Fats.

From Chapter 28, we can summarize the different Fats as follows:

> **Monounsaturated Fats** – These are regarded as healthy fats for good reasons. The Monounsaturated Fat Oleic Acid is the main fat used by the body both for energy and to store energy.
>
> **Polyunsaturated Fats** – These are essential nutrients. Rather than being key energy nutrients, they provide a host of wider health benefits. We have covered these in some detail already.
>
> But it is worth noting again that new seed-based oils such as Sunflower Oil, or Rapeseed (Canola) oil, have a high Omega 6 content and do need to be treated with a bit of caution.
>
> **Saturated Fats** – These have been much maligned, but it turns out that we do need some of these fats in our diet.
>
> The mixed messages regarding these Fats is highlighted by the way that the Medium Chain Fatty Acids, or MCTs found in

various plant foods such coconuts, are deemed to be healthy, and yet those same MCTs found in Dairy Foods are not.

It does appear that many issues relating to our diet are nuanced. We all have to explore the options that suit our preferences, our budgets and our own likes and dislikes.

Trans Fats and Hydrogenated Oils – Now we know that the natural Trans Fats found in small quantities in some Meat Foods are not really an issue, but we do need to be wary of the man-made Trans Fats.

This can be problematic because they are used for all sorts of food production. We can all treat these with a bit of caution and find alternatives if we can.

I am aware that I need something like 3 ½ oz of Fats in my daily diet, and sometimes more when I am very active. So, the issue is not about cutting them out but maintaining a balance across the whole spectrum of Fats. For example, I happily include Saturated Fats, not just for the energy, but for the Vitamins and Minerals too. But I also make sure not to include excessive amounts.

However, I take a more cautious approach with the man-made Trans Fats. Studying my own diet, I found these were usually occurring in Pastries, Prepared Puddings and Prepared Meals.

As it happens, I rarely eat "prepared foods" from the supermarket, and I treat Pastries and Puddings as "once in a while treats". This means that my regular diet isn't loaded with hidden extras.

If I do eat a prepared meal, and my local supermarket does offer some very delectable "prepared dishes", then it's like my Puddings, I can enjoy them from time to time knowing that they are part of weekly diet plan that has fueled me up for life.

In fact, rather than worrying about my fats I look at them as a source of key vitamins and minerals as well as being a key energy food too.

A Completely New Outlook on my Food

But the most exciting outcome of all was that I found myself looking at and planning my food, not on what to leave out or cut down on, but always trying to work out:

What foods to include to cover all my nutrients and provide the optimum amount of energy.

Rather than worrying if I have included too much Fat in my meal plan, I'm checking to see if I have covered my Omega 3s, especially my DHA and EPA, and included some Omega 6. And that I have kept the Trans Fats to the absolute minimum or excluded them altogether.

I have already covered my Fibres, Antioxidants, Phytochemicals, Prebiotics and Probiotics as well as my Proteins using Diet Hacks 1 and 2. I have topped up my Carbs, so now I can make sure I am covering all my Vitamins and Minerals too.

Which brings me back to processed foods which includes the foods in the bottom half of Table 20. You see the mix of carbs and fats in so many processed foods that line the supermarket shelves really hits a lot of our sensory triggers. And don't the food companies know it.

But now confronted with a burning desire to eat a whole lot of junk or not, I find myself asking:

"Who's in charge here, Me or the Food Company?"

I still enjoy that feeling of putting the offending item back on the shelf and moving on in search of foods that will genuinely nourish me.

A New Look at Food Plates

Early in this Chapter I told you of my surprise at just how modest my portions of Concentrated Carb Foods became and the easiest way to describe this is through the evolution of my own "Food Plate".

Now different organizations present "Food Plates" or "Plates of Food" which may go hand in hand with their respective "Food Pyramids". We'll start with the plates and cover the pyramids in the following Chapter.

I tend to eat a main meal in the evening, and I just got into the habit of measuring out my Concentrated Carbs last. After trial and error over many months, I found the "Plate Portions" shown in the left column of Table 28 opposite worked best for me.

If I was burning up a lot of calories through extra activities, then I might eat a bit more. But even so, I was genuinely surprised at how modest the portions were and yet they certainly fueled me up for life. That continues to this day.

My Food Plate	Canada's Food Plate
½ plate non-starchy vegies and/or salad **1/3** plate protein portion **1/6** plate starchy carb or other energy foods like rice or quinoa or legumes	½ plate vegies and fruit ¼ plate protein foods ¼ plate whole grain foods

Table 28 Comparing Food Plates

I quickly found, and still find, that if I eat too much of my Concentrated Carbs then I quickly feel bloated rather than satiated or satisfied. But I am aware that we all have to find what works for us.

Now comparing my own Food Plate with others is interesting. For example, the "Canada's Food Plate" described in more detail on the Government of Canada website, **(Online Source 41),** is also shown in Table 28.

If you follow the link to their website, you will see that "Canada's Food Guide" include the Starchy vegetables together with some Legumes in their ½ plate of veggies and fruit.

However, as we covered again earlier in this Chapter, the different Food Groups are organized into 4 Categories. Category 3 includes the high energy Starchy Veggies paired with the high energy Grains and their Derivatives, as shown in Table 10.

I refer to Category 3 as my "Concentrated Carbs" and these are the high energy foods that I include in that modest 1/6 plate. But don't forget even these small portions still pack a lot of calories!

Conversely, I aim to only include Non-Starchy veggies in my **½ plate,** but sometimes might include peas, which are Legumes of course, or sweetcorn. I just happen to like peas, and I might include sweetcorn if I am low on other veggies. But the overall aim is to focus on Non-Starchy veggies.

The "Canada's Food Plate" does illustrate the tendency of many health organizations to recommend higher levels of "Grains" in the regular diet. But we must also consider the following:

1. "Food Plates" are often trying to capture all the food for the day rather than just 1 meal
2. If you follow a vegetarian or vegan diet you might well include more grains and legumes as part of your protein foods

On the first point I would emphasize that my own "Food Plate" is my ideal main meal and is part of the overall food for the day.

And on this second point you will recall this observation about wheat from Chapter 24:

> ...according to the International Development Research Centre, IDRC, wheat "provides more calories and protein in the world's diet than any other crop".

Whilst I include Category 3 foods from Table 10 for the energy they provide, they also provide diversity to help to cover all my amino acids.

But, if you are following a vegetarian or vegan diet and including more "Grains", "Legumes & Pseudo Cereals" and "Tree Nuts & Seeds" as your key Protein foods, then you must take into account the high energy content accompanying these particular Foods.

Whilst I find the concept of the "Food Plate" useful for my main meal, it does have limitations when used to try and represent all my food intake across a whole day.

Revisiting the Daily Protein Intake Chart

In the end I found the Daily Protein Intake Chart was the easiest tool to represent my overall daily food, and especially after I added the extra column for "**Veg, Salad & Fruit**", as in Tables 24, which is shown again on the page opposite.

	My Proteins	1. Total Protein content	BV (%)	2. Total Absorbed Proteins	Veg, Salad & Fruit
Morning Starter					Small portion of fruit Satsuma
Breakfast	2 Med eggs 2 slice of whole grain toast Greek style Yoghurt	12g 8g 13g	93.7 64 84	11.2g 5.1g 10.9g	
Lunch	1 oz grilled chicken breast 2 slices of whole grain bread Sprinkle of seeds	8.2g 8g 2g	74 64 70	6.1g 5.1g 1.4g	Stuff the sandwich with loads of salad
Post Exercise Snack	Glass of milk Handful of Cashew & Brazil nuts	8g 5g	84.5 60	6.8g 3g	Eat a Banana a little later
Dinner or Evening Meal	4 oz fish/meat ¼ cup Quinoa	34.6g 5.5g	74.3 83	25.7g 4.7g	My ½ plate of non-starchy veggies Or Plate of salad
Total Proteins		**104.3g**		**80.0g**	
My Average RDA of Reference Proteins				**74.8g**	
Average Biological Value of Total Daily Proteins		**80/104.3**	**=**	**77%**	

Table 24 (Again) Calculating My Daily Protein Intake

I still use my Food Plate to plan my main meal, or rather the portion sizes of my non-starchy veggies and to remind myself how little Concentrated Carbs I need. In fact some days I might cut out that "¼ cup Quinoa" if I don't really need the Concentrated Carbs.

The important point here is that by taking everything back to the Base Nutrients, our Food Types, then just about anyone can adapt the Food Groups and Categories, the Food Plate and the Daily Protein Intake Chart to suit their food preferences or tastes or budgets.

Now because I am happy to include Meat, Fish, Dairy and Eggs it is quite easy to cover my Protein requirements and especially cover all the Amino Acids. So, the Daily Protein Intake Chart helps me maintain and encourage diversity in order to also cover the extra vitamins, minerals and other nutrients these important foods contain.

But for Sue, the chart primarily serves more as a reminder of how carefully she needs to plan her Proteins, as presented in Tables 25, which is shown again on the page opposite.

Now she is following a vegetarian diet which includes dairy products and eggs. For anyone following a vegan diet, the need to balance their full Protein requirements with the extra energy from Grains, Pseudo-Grains, Legumes, Tree Nuts and Seeds becomes more challenging.

Making it Work by Making it Simple

Finally, using this simple meal planning process means that I am in control of my diet and my calories without really trying.

I find this still works even if my meal plan is just literally sketching in a preferred choice of proteins and some veggie ideas depending on what I have already or what I can then buy, or a particular dish I might like to prepare.

Indeed, over time I found myself just mapping out my meals in my head. I might double check my Protein Count from time to time, but the 3 Diet Hacks quickly became just regular habits.

Now you have a few tools to help you experiment with your diet to find what works best for you. And there is one more tool you might find useful, the "Food Pyramid", which we cover in the next Chapter.

	Sue's Proteins	**1. Total Protein content**	**BV (%)**	**2. Total Absorbed Proteins**	**Veg, Salad & Fruit**
Morning Starter					
Breakfast	1/3 cup Greek Style Yoghurt Corn Flakes	4.3g 2g	84 (65)	3.6g 1.3g	
Lunch	Egg Mayo Sandwich Filling 2 slices of whole grain bread Sprinkle of seeds	3g 8g 2g	93.7 64 70	2.8g 5.1g 1.4g	
Light Snack					
Dinner or Evening Meal	3 oz Tofu ¼ cup Legumes Handful of nuts	14.5g 4g 5g	74 68 60	10.7g 2.7g 3g	
Total Proteins		**42.8g**		**30.6g**	
Sue's Average RDA of Reference Proteins				**39.6g**	
Average Biological Value of Total Daily Proteins		**30.6/42.8**	**=**	**71.4%**	

Table 25 (Again) Calculating Sue's Daily Protein Intake

35. Diet Hacks, Food Pyramids and My Small Intestines

I started using the original 3 Guidelines all those years ago to recover from a serious illness. But having got my diet back in order and regained "reasonable" health again I stupidly let it all slip away. The really daft thing was that I was so busy looking after everyone else's diets, I didn't look after my own.

When I did start to look after myself properly again in 2013, I had a nagging fear or suspicion that if I over complicated things, I would end up letting it slip away again. I had to do things differently.

I didn't want my framework to be a battle of discipline or willpower. I didn't want it to be rigid or restrictive. I was desperate to make my food fun, enjoyable and so easy that I would now stick to it for life.

So, I stripped everything back to the base nutrients, went back to what worked and reviewed that in the light of the emerging science which has moved forward in leaps and bounds over the last twenty-five years or so. I refined my nutrition down to 3 simple diet hacks which provide a framework that I still follow to this day. And we have covered these in some detail:

> **Diet Hack 1** - Eat a variety of fresh non-starchy veg & salad in 4 generous portions and fruit in modest portions – Food Priority 1.
>
> **Diet Hack 2** - Count my proteins (and include a wide variety) – Food Priority 2.
>
> **Diet Hack 3** - Plan my meals (to cover my optimum energy calories each day) – Food Priorities 3-6.

Then I set out to build my own "Food Pyramid" to go with the simple visual guides like my "Daily Protein Intake Chart" and "Food Plate".

I have always liked the concept of the "Food Pyramid". So, I set about developing my own modified version to provide a simple overview of all my food choices and to help me include as much food diversity as possible, in roughly the right relative amounts.

And I suggest that you try it out as well. Yours will be different to mine, I'm sure, but that is the point. We all have our own individual tastes, preferences, budgets and so on, but we still all need to find the same base nutrients in roughly the right proportions to suit our individual requirements.

But maybe I should start with some background on this great tool.

The Early Food Pyramids with an Emphasis on Grains

In 1974 Anna-Britt Agnsäter, an educator working for a Swedish grocery cooperative developed what is generally recognised as the first Food Pyramid, **(Online Source 42)**.

The main Food Groups recommended for a healthy diet were arranged within a pyramid shape. Those foods we need to eat more of formed the base and foods we needed less of were higher up the pyramid.

I should point out that there was quite an emphasis on Grains which formed the base of the pyramid.

Then in 1992 the US government developed the Food Pyramid Guide in conjunction with the Harvard School of Public Health. And again, there was quite an emphasis on grains, even going so far as to recommend 5 servings of Grains a day.

This idea evolved over time and in the US the Harvard School of Public Health working in conjunction with the USDA developed the concept of the "My.Pyramid" and the "Healthy Eating Plate". Here in the UK the NHS developed and promoted the "Eat Well Plate".

All these sources have some merit; however, there seemed to be a trend to place considerable emphasis on Grains in the diet. This emphasis on Grains does continue to some degree as we saw with the "Canada's Food Plate" in the previous Chapter. And this was highlighted back in

Chapter 19 where I quoted an article from University of California, San Francisco in which they suggest:

- As a general rule, include at least one serving of whole grain in every meal.

Indeed, one of the latest Food Pyramids proposed by the Harvard T.H. Chan School of Public Health (renamed in 2014) continues this emphasis. They provide an excellent downloadable handout via their website, **(Online Source 43).** Interestingly, this latest version starts with:

Daily Exercise & Weight Control

This message forms the very base of the pyramid, and the same downloadable handout expands on this with the following:

START WITH EXERCISE

A healthy diet is built on a base of regular exercise, which keeps calories in balance and weight in check. Be physically active. Any activity is better than none. And more is usually better.

Well, I am all for Daily Exercise. As for the Weight Control, I prefer to think of this as an outcome from a combination of a sensible diet and being "physically active".

This addition to the Food Pyramid does convey the really important message that:

The Human Body is Designed to Move

I will come back to this shortly, but first I will run through the evolution of my own Food Pyramid.

My Small Intestines and the Base of My Pyramid

As I started to dabble with my own Food Pyramid, I thought that maybe my circumstances were not widely applicable. After all, at the outset of my journey I was struggling from the effects of a severe tropical illness, my small intestines were barely functioning, and I was living off pills and shakes.

Much as I might have wanted to build regular exercise back into my life, I was in such poor shape that it was a problem. My immediate problem was finding a way to get my small intestines working again.

Through trial and error, I found that including a selection of Non-Starchy Veggies and some Fruit every day made a huge difference. I adopted the "5 a Day" approach and the benefits followed.

Naturally life got in the way, and from time to time I wavered from the approach over the years. Every time I let it slip; I suffered the consequences. But every time I re-adopted the "5 a Day" approach the positive impact on my own health and fitness was dramatic.

As my 3 Diet Hacks were crystallising, I realised that the Non-Starchy Veggies and Fruits in my "5 a Day" were the stars of my diet. In fact:

> **Everything in my diet now started with a selection of 4 generous portions of fresh non-starchy vegetables and salads, plus modest portions of fruit.**

I came to realise that these are the foods that provide:

- Many of our vitamins and minerals,
- The bulk of our soluble and insoluble fibres to help our digestive system work efficiently,
- The prebiotics for our gut flora
- The antioxidants to help our lymphatic and cardiovascular systems flush the waste products from our muscles and organs
- The multitude of phytochemicals that help regulate so many of the processes in the body
- Some of the slow-release energy that also helps satiate

Phew! That's quite a list.

In fact, they formed the base of my own Food Pyramid which is shown in **Fig 14** shortly. They were the foundation that helped get my small intestines working properly again and gave me my life back. But there is something else. It is difficult to explain, and this may be just me.

I might be particularly aware of my digestive system, more so than most perhaps. This is probably the result of knowing what it's like when it isn't working, especially my small intestine.

When I get my "5 a Day" more or less right, then it's like the small intestines are "purring". Conversely, when I get out of kilter, I can feel everything grinding to a halt.

And I suspect that one overlooked factor may be the role of both the Insoluble Fibres and Soluble Fibres in creating the optimum viscosity of the Chyme. Get this about right and the food passing from the stomach and into the small intestine is well prepared for the journey through the remarkable physical complexity created by the folded mucosa, as described back in Chapter 16.

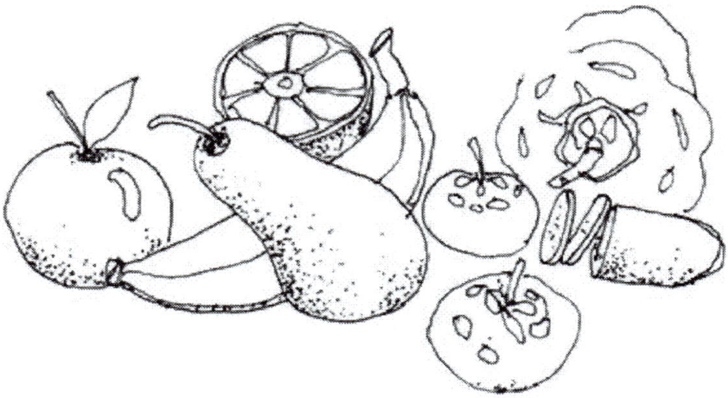

Fig 10. The stars of your diet ***(Repeat from page 205)***

In addition, as we become more aware of the role our Gut Flora plays, we are able to positively impact on that delicate balance between good microbes and the bad microbes that is such an important part of the human condition. This is such an exciting area of our diet.

So, for me, the non-starchy veggies and fruits aren't just the Stars of My Diet, they form the broad base of my own Food Pyramid, the foundation if you like. And maybe instead of the call for "Daily Exercise & Weight Control", I should start with a call to:

Look after your Gut & your Gut Flora

And I will come back to Exercise shortly.

A Caveat and Why We All need to Experiment.

There are some specific populations and diets around the world where the "5 A Day" rule doesn't really apply. The Inuit of North America are one such example. The extreme climate is not conducive to much plant life suitable for human consumption and as a result they have developed a very specialised diet.

But this is an exception and might only apply to a small percentage of the whole world population. Whereas, for those of us brought up with a Modern Farmer Diet in one guise or another, I would suggest that the advice from WHO may be applicable to most of us to some degree.

Even so, we must all experiment to find what works best for each of us. The portions sizes that work for me may be a bit larger than most.

You might even find that using foods like Legumes or Pseudo-Cereals for some of your "5 a Day" requirement works for you. Either way, you now have the tools to experiment to find what works best for you.

Proteins and Food Preferences

Our Proteins present a different challenge or rather set of challenges. We can all be a bit blasé about our Proteins, but the reality is that we should consider them carefully:

- Am I eating enough Protein?
- Am I eating too much Protein?
- Am I covering the full range of Amino Acids?

The surprising thing about our Proteins, or rather the constituent Amino Acids, is just how efficiently the body uses them.

It doesn't matter what your food preferences are, we can all make a reasonable estimate of our adequate protein intake and then make a good estimate of an optimal level averaged out over a few days or even a week. This helps simplify meal planning.

We can use the Food Pyramid to gauge roughly how much of the different Protein foods we eat relative to other foods and how much energy is combined with the different Food Groups.

Our Genuine Energy Requirements

There is a point I keep coming back to and that is:

> **Many of the new foods in the Modern Farmer Diet are packed with energy. It is very easy to just eat too much energy.**

My comments about grains are not to criticise them as a valuable food, but to highlight that sometimes we forget how efficiently the body digests and absorbs the energy.

We humans have produced all sorts of wonderful foods, but the goal here is to maximise the benefit of all these wonderful foods. As a result, our high energy foods sit surprisingly high up the Pyramid.

A New Food Pyramid

The purpose of the Food Pyramid is to provide a visual picture of all the different foods you can pick and choose from to include in your diet and a rough guide to relative amounts of the different foods.

My own version is shown in **Fig 14** on the following page. The non-starchy vegetables and salads are the foundation of my diet and form the base of this Pyramid.

Although we only need modest amounts of fruit, their position reflects their role as part of the foundation and the effort it takes to maintain a diverse and regular selection in the diet.

Above the Fruit, the pyramid reflects the amount or volume of the different food that we need. So, as you move up the pyramid, you can pick and choose from all the different foods depending on your own preferences.

This is subjective of course. I'm trying to cater for a couple of omnivores, a discerning carnivore, a vegetarian who eats occasional fish and a vegetarian who does eat dairy and eggs. But we manage to cover all our bases.

If your preference is to follow a stricter vegetarian or vegan diet, then you can pick and choose accordingly. Likewise, if you are strictly carnivore or pescatarian.

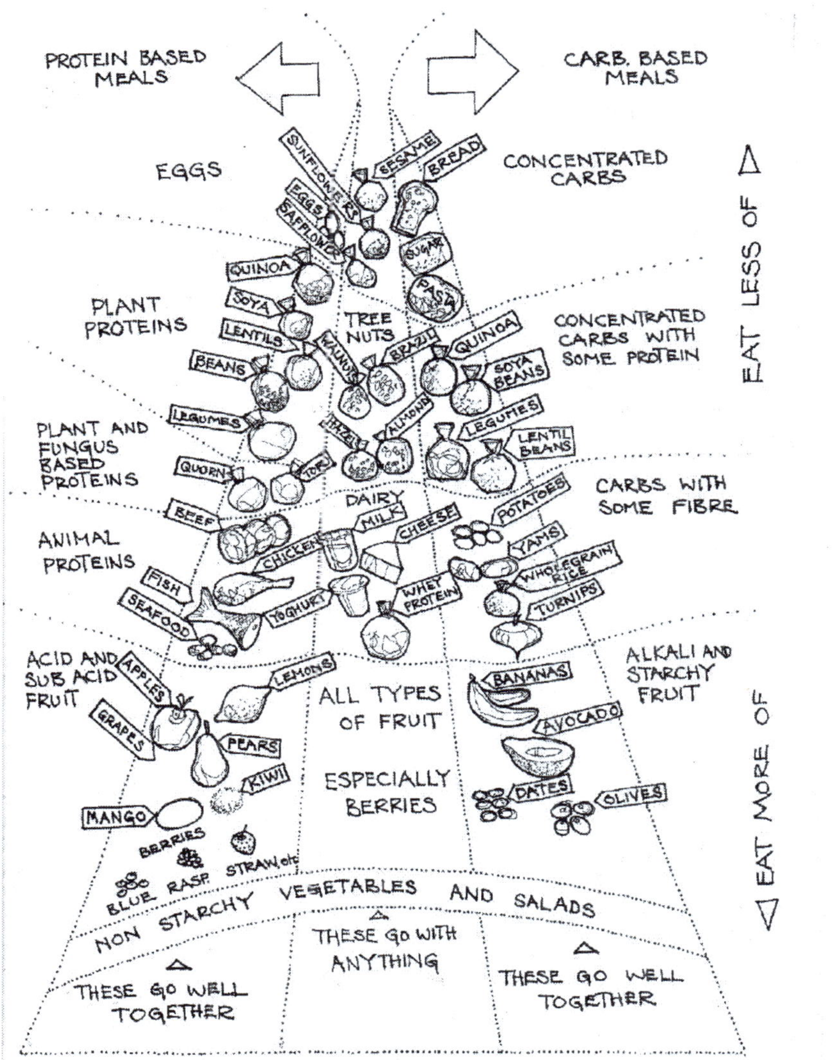

Look after your Gut & your Gut Flora

Fig 16. A Different Take on The Food Pyramid

As you use the Food Pyramid you quickly become aware of which foods you can eat more of and which foods you should maybe eat a little less of.

And in the fullness of time, you might progress to planning meals with an emphasis on fats and carbs for energy or proteins for rebuilding muscle, which we can cover in the next book.

But for now, just try building your own Food Pyramid. Play around with it. You might find it gives you a few pointers as to how you can start modifying your current diet straight away. And you can use it to explore new food options.

Remember your food should be fun and enjoyable, an adventure even.

Health & Fitness and your Diet

When the Harvard T.H. Chan School of Public Health published their downloadable handout via their website, **(Online Source 43)**, I thought they were really onto something.

I couldn't agree more that health and fitness are interlinked and that they are both underpinned by your diet. But there is something even more fundamental in this message and it is that:

The Human Body is Designed to Move

We are not designed to be sitting around idly all day; we are designed for movement. I talked about our two "Energy Batteries" but more interestingly we have three main energy systems that enable us to operate at different levels of intensity. But we must activate these systems get the most from them.

Our bones and joints are designed get stronger with impact. It is sitting around that makes them weak and brittle. Our heart and cardiovascular system get stronger with exercise. On and on goes the list of benefits.

But I do understand that this seems beyond many of us, so I will cover how putting my own diet in order encouraged me to get active again in the closing Chapter. And if I could get moving again, then just about anybody can.

36. Building "A Diet You Can Live With"

A couple of simple steps to get you started

One key aim of this book is to encourage you to explore the food choices you already make so you can start to appreciate how many of your nutrients you are already including. Then you can get a feel for where you can improve your diet.

Feel free to use Table 29 below to start recording the foods you already eat and foods you would like to include in your new diet.

But rather than me giving you endless lists of Foods in the different Food Groups, I have included a modest selection to provide a springboard to explore your current choices. There are also a few extra pages for any notes you might want to make.

I would also add that if you choose not to eat foods from a Food Group such as "Meat, Fish & Eggs" for example, that's fine, just explore the groups you prefer. You'll notice that I have highlighted both the Fruits and Non-Starchy Vegetables.

I would like to suggest that in particular you use Table 29 to jot down the fruits, non-starchy vegetables and salads you already include. And if you run out of space, make a second copy to jot down the Fruits and Non-Starchy Vegetables you would like to include in your regular diet.

And use Table 30 to start building a list of your Protein Foods and their Biological Values to calculate the protein in your regular portions.

There is also a simple website where you can download copies of the various Food Tables and Planners which you can find at:

www.adietyoucanlivewith.com

This book is intended to start you on a journey of exploration, but I appreciate that it might still seem daunting, especially with regard to the proteins. Part of that might be a result of the shifting food preferences across many societies today.

The main thing is to start thinking of your protein foods in terms of the base nutrients, the constituent Amino Acids, that we all need. And please remember that this is just the start. If you are interested, we go into a lot more detail on the Biological Value of different proteins and ways to measure how much protein in regular portions in Book 2.

Food Preferences or Finding What Works for You?

At the outset I suggested that just about anyone can use the framework and the 3 Diet Hacks, even across a range of food preferences including omnivores, vegetarians and vegans.

However, the real aim of the book is to encourage you to explore your own diet and find what works for you. I am quite happy that everyone should choose their own foods based on their own tastes, budgets and values, but at the end of the day the key to a healthy diet is that you include all the nutrients you need in roughly the right amounts and proportions in foods that you are able to fully digest.

All I can suggest is that you try to read beyond the headlines. Just about everything to do with diet is nuanced. What works for one person, might not work for another. And just because one person chooses to follow one particular food preference doesn't mean everyone else has to follow. You need all your nutrients and hopefully this book helps you along the way to building the best diet possible for you.

My biggest hope is that you:

Start experimenting with your food to find what works best for you

As for my own journey, well I was staring at a life fueled by shakes and pills. My small intestines didn't work, and I struggled to digest and absorb most nutrients. But using the framework and 3 Diet Hacks I can follow an omnivore diet enjoying my "real" food and enjoying good health and fitness as a result. Where will your journey take you?

Getting Active Again

There is one more thing. As I set out to rebuild my diet, I also wanted to build activity back into my life. As my energy returned, I tried exercising, but all I could manage was a brisk walk. So, I started walking. I even devised simple routines that helped me fire up all three energy systems. It worked so well that I qualified as a Firefighter @56. You can find how at:

www.walkruntrain.com

Don't underestimate the power of walking, it could just turn things around for you. It certainly worked for me.

Ready to move on?

Enough of the Why. If you are ready to start exploring your food options armed with the new insights presented here, then:

Let's start building a diet to power you up for life

And if you are not active already, then you might find yourself so full of energy that you just have to start doing something.

As you start getting active again, you may well find that you just want to eat better to power up your day. And as you power up your day you just want to get even more active.

Before you know it, you'll be off hiking that trail you always wanted to hike or taking on your first 5k run for the fun of it or heading back to the gym again. All powered by your new diet:

A Diet You Can Live With

Food Group	Examples	Foods I Eat	Frequency
Meat, Fish and Eggs	Beef, chicken, pork, game, cod, salmon, crab, eggs		
Concentrated plant/fungus protein	Tofu. Quorn, Tempeh		
Tree Nuts and Seeds	Walnuts, Brazil Nuts, Cashew, Sesame, Flax, Sunflower		
Legumes and Pseudo-cereals	Lentils, Peas, beans, peanuts, chickpeas, quinoa, buckwheat,		
Grains and derivatives	Wheat, spelt oats, rice, bread, pasta,		
Starchy vegetables	Potatoes, yams, carrots, parsnips, sweet corn		
Fruits	Apples, pears, plums, oranges, peaches, mango, berries, bananas		
Non-starchy vegetables salads, mushrooms	Cabbage, kale, broccoli, spinach cauliflower, peppers, lettuce, radish, onions, garlic mushrooms,		
Milk & Dairy	Milk, yoghurt, cheese, cottage cheese, butter,		

Table 29 The Foods you eat Regularly.

Protein Food	Typical Portion	Gram of Protein /typical portion	Estimated Biological Value %	Gram of Protein actually absorbed

TABLE 30 The Biological Value of your Protein foods

	My Proteins	Protein content	BV (%)	Absorbed Proteins	Veg, Salad & Fruit
Morning Starter					
Breakfast					
Lunch					
Post Exercise Snack					
Dinner or Evening Meal					
Total Proteins		**g**		**g**	
My RDA of Reference Proteins				**g**	
Average Biological Value of Total Daily Proteins				**%**	

Table 27 Blank Table to Calculate Your Daily Protein page 238

Notes

37. References, Online Sources and Downloads

References

Ref 1 (Page 19) - Cathy O'Neil (2016) *Weapons of Math Destruction, How big data increases inequality and threatens democracy*. 1st edn. London: Penguin

Ref 2 (Page 20) - Elizabeth Blackburn and Elissa Epel (2017) *The Telomere Effect, A revolutionary approach to living younger, healthier, longer*. 1st edn. London: Orion Spring

Ref 3 (Page 39 & 136) - Christopher Westhorp (2017), *The Commando Packet Manual 1940-1945,* Osprey Publishing

Ref 4 (Page 45 & 158) – Brad Pilon (Copyright © 2008-2011) – *How Much Protein*, by Strength Works, Inc.

Ref 5 (Page 49 & 244)– Lawrence Alderson (1994) *The Chance to Survive*, 2nd revised edn, Pilkington Press Limited. See page 86

Ref 6 (Page 52, 56 & 246) – Jane Higdon (2003) *An Evidence-based Approach to Vitamins and Minerals: Health Benefits and Intake Recommendations*, 1st edn. Published by Thieme.

Ref 7 (Page 75)– Philip Walling (2018) *Till the cows come home.* 1st edn, Atlantic Books, an Imprint of Atlantis Books Ltd, London.

Ref 8 (Page 77)– Catherine Rogers (2019) *Gut Well Soon,* Panoma Press, St Albans, Herts.

Ref 9 (Page 98)– Jayne Buxton (2022) *The Great Plant-Based Con,* Piatkus, London.

Ref 10 (Page 98)– T. Colin Campbell, PhD and Thomas M. Campbell (2006) *The China Study,* BenBella Books, Inc, Dallas, TX.

Ref 11 (Page 124 & 219) – Prof Richard Wrangham (2010) – *Catching Fire – How cooking made us human*, 1st Paperback edn, Profile Books Ltd.

Ref 12 (Page 157)- Diana Rogers and Robb Wolf (Copyright © 2020) – *The Sacred Cow*, BenBella Books, Inc, Dallas, TX.

Personal Discussions

Ref A (Page 137) – Toby Garbett, Toby kindly discussed aspects of Nutrition and Training from his time with the GB Rowing Squad. You can find out more about Toby's successful rowing career and his successful business career in the Health & Fitness domain by visiting his website:

<https://tggymwellness.com/personal-training/toby-garbett/>

Online Sources

Source 1 (Page 19) – *Measuring the Waist* by The World Cancer Research Fund <https://www.wcrf-uk.org/uk/here-help/health-tools/how-to-measure-your-waist>.

Source 2 (Page 21) – *Nutrition in the Prevention and Treatment of Abdominal Obesity* (Second Edition), 2019, by Alaa Youssef Ahmed Ahmed Baioumi (Now you have to pay for the PDF, unfortunately) <https://www.sciencedirect.com/science/article/abs/pii/B9780128 160930000033>

Source 3 (Page 39) – The Faculty of Public Health n.d., *Dietary Reference Values (DRVs), current dietary goals, recommendations, guidelines and the evidence for them,* on the Health Knowledge website, <https://www.healthknowledge.org.uk/public-health-textbook/disease-causation-diagnostic/2e-health-social-behaviour/drvs>

Source 4 (Page 43) – Genetic Science Learning Center, n.d., University of Utah, *9 Types of Proteins,* Online information page published by the Genetic Science Learning Center on their Learn.Genetics website, <https://learn.genetics.utah.edu/content/evolution/proteintypes >.

Source 5 (Page 48) – Micronutrient Information Centre, n.d., *Essential Fatty Acids*, Linus Pauling Institute, Oregon State University, <https://lpi.oregonstate.edu/mic/other-nutrients/essential-fatty-acids>

Source 6 (Page 49 & 170) – Danielle Swanson, Robert Block and Shaker A. Mousa, American Society for Nutrition (2012), *Omega-3 Fatty-Acids EPA and DHA: Health Benefits Throughout Life*, The

National Center for Biotechnology Information website, <https://www.ncbi.nlm.nih.gov/pmc/articles/PMC3262608/>

Source 7 (Page 51) – George T. Griffing, MD, Professor of Medicine, Editor in Chief (2008), *Mother Was Right About Cod-Liver Oil,* the Medscape Journal of Medicine, <https://www.ncbi.nlm.nih.gov/pmc/articles/PMC2258476/>

Source 8 (Page 52) – National Research Council (US) Committee on Diet and Health (DC), (1989), *Diet and Health Implications for Reducing Chronic Disease Risk,* National Academies Press (US) <https://www.ncbi.nlm.nih.gov/books/NBK218756/>

<https://www.ncbi.nlm.nih.gov/books/NBK218749/>

Source 9 (Page 54, 209 & 235) – Stephen Walsh, a Vegan Society trustee, and other members of the International Vegetarian Union Science Group (IVU-SCI), (October 2001), *What Every Vegan Should Know About Vitamin B12*, on the Vegan Society website, <https://www.vegansociety.com/resources/nutrition-and-health/nutrients/vitamin-b12/what-every-vegan-should-know-about-vitamin-b12>

Source 10 (Page 56) – My Health Alberta, March 2023), *Minerals: Their Functions and Sources,* My Health Alberta website, <https://myhealth.alberta.ca/health/Pages/conditions.aspx?hwid=ta3912&>

Source 11 (Page 56) – Micronutrient Information Center, n.d., *Minerals*, Linus Pauling Institute, Oregon State University, <https://lpi.oregonstate.edu/mic/minerals>

Source 12 (Page 66) – Katherine McManus, MS, RD, LDN, (2019), *Should I be eating more fiber?* Harvard Health Blog,

<https://www.health.harvard.edu/blog/should-i-be-eating-more-fiber-2019022115927>

Source 13 (Page 71 & 85) – Patient Education at The University of California San Francisco, n.d., *Increasing Fiber Intake*, University of California San Francisco, <https://www.ucsfhealth.org/education/increasing-fiber-intake>

<https://uhs.berkeley.edu/sites/default/files/dietaryfiber.pdf>

Source 14 (Page 73) – Susan L. Prescott, (2017), *History of medicine. Origin of the term microbiome and why it matters,* the Human Microbiome Journal on The Elsevier ScienceDirect website. <https://www.sciencedirect.com/science/article/pii/S24522317173 0012X#b0105>

Source 15 (Page 74) – Elizabeth Thursby and Nathalie Juge; (2017), *Introduction to the human gut microbiome,* Published in the Biochemical Journal and the National Library of Medicine, on the National Center for Biotechnology Information website. <https://www.ncbi.nlm.nih.gov/pmc/articles/PMC5433529/>

Source 16 (Page 80) – Reviewed by Stacy Sampson, D.O. and by Jamie Eske, (2019), *How does oxidative stress affect the body?*

Reviewed by Rose Wilson, Ph.D., MSN, R.N., IBCLC, AHN-BC, CHT and Zawn Villines, (2019), *How do free radicals affect the body?*

Both articles on Medical News Today, <https://www.medicalnewstoday.com/articles/324863>

Source 17 (Page 80) – Jennifer Weinberg, *Revitalize Your Lymphatic System for Clearer Skin, Vibrant Energy & More Efficient Metabolism*, on her dedicated Website,

<https://www.jenniferweinbergmd.com/revitalize-your-lymphatic-system/>

Source 18 (Page 82 & 93) – Emilia Klapp, n.d, *Types of Phytochemicals,* on the Share.com website, <https://www.sharecare.com/health/nutrition-diet/types-of-phytochemicals>

Source 19 (Page 82) – Nicolas Monjotin, Marie Josèphe Amiot, Jacques Fleurentin, Jean Michel Morel, Sylvie Raynal, (2022), *Clinical Evidence of the Benefits of Phytonutrients in Human Healthcare*, the National Library of Medicine on the National Center for Biotechnology Information website, <https://pmc.ncbi.nlm.nih.gov/articles/PMC9102588/>

Source 20 (Page 88) – Jillian Levy, (2022), *15 Fermented Foods for a Healthy Gut and Overall Health*, Dr. Axe website, <https://draxe.com/nutrition/fermented-foods/>

Source 21 (Page 89) – Arlene Semeco, MS, RD and Erin Kelly and medically reviewed by Amy Richter, RD, Nutrition, (2023), *The 19 Best Prebiotic Foods You Should Eat*, on the Healthline website, <https://www.healthline.com/nutrition/19-best-prebiotic-foods>

Source 22 (Page 90) – Zawn Villines and medically reviewed by Hope Warshaw, R.D., CDE, (2019) *What are the worst foods for gut health?* On the Medical News Today website, <https://www.medicalnewstoday.com/articles/326256.php>

Source 23 (Page 92 & 101) – S. Bengmark, n.d. *The "new" lifestyle—a threat to health?* on the Lund University Publications website. Sadly Prof. Stig Bengmark passed away in Dec 2023, but his legacy lives on through the company Synbiotics AB, at < https://stigbengmark.com/en/ >

Source 24 (Page 96) – Balz Frei, Emeritus Professor at Oregon State University, (2007), *Studies Force New View on Biology, Nutritional Action of Flavonoids*, on the Newsroom website for Oregon State University, <https://today.oregonstate.edu/archives/2007/mar/studies-force-new-view-biology-nutritional-action-flavonoids>

Source 25 (Page 111) – Kaitlyn Berkheiser and medically reviewed by Jillian Kubala, MS, RD, Nutrition, (2019), *What's the Difference Between Tempeh and Tofu?* On the Healthline website, <https://www.healthline.com/nutrition/tempeh-vs-tofu>.

Source 26 (Page 112) – Kris Gunnars, BSc, and medically reviewed by Kim Chin, RD, Nutrition, (2023), *How to Optimize Your Omega-6 to Omega-3 Ratio*, On the Healthline website, <https://www.healthline.com/nutrition/optimize-omega-6-omega-3-ratio#section3>

Source 27 (Page 113) – Lizzie Streit, MS, RDN, LD and Ruairi Robertson, PhD and medically reviewed by Adrienne Seitz, MS, RD, LDN, Nutrition, (2023), *9 Healthy Beans and Legumes You Should Try*, on the Healthline website,

<https://www.healthline.com/nutrition/healthiest-beans-legumes#section2>

Source 28 (Page 114) – International Development Research Centre, (IDRC), Canada, (2010), *Facts & Figures on Food and Biodiversity*, on the IDRC-CRDI website, <https://idrc-crdi.ca/en/research-in-action/facts-figures-food-and-biodiversity>

Source 29 (Page 124) – Nutri Advanced, (2017), *Did Omega-3 Shape the History of the Human Race?* on the Nutri Advanced website, <https://www.nutriadvanced.co.uk/news/did-omega-3-shape-the-history-of-the-human-race/>

Source 30 (Page 128) – John Koster, (2024), *Mago of Carthage is the Father of Agriculture and Farming,* on the PhoeniciaOrg website, <https://phoenicia.org/Mago-Carthage-Father-of-Agriculture.html>

Source 31 (Page 135) – UN News, (2022), Once again, *US and Europe way ahead on daily calorie intake*, on the UN News website, <https://news.un.org/en/story/2022/12/1131637>

Source 32 (Page 151) – National Research Council (US), (1989), *Recommended Dietary Allowances, 10th Edition,* National Library of Medicine on the National Center for Biotechnology Information website, <https://www.ncbi.nlm.nih.gov/books/NBK234932/>

Source 33 (Page 151) – Prepared for the Department of Health by Jenny Salmon BS c MSc (Nutrition), (1991), *Dietary Reference Values A Guide*, on the UK Government website, <https://assets.publishing.service.gov.uk/media/5bab995240f0b607130bd49d/Dietary_Reference_Values_-_A_Guide__1991_.pdf>

Source 34 (Page 166) – Atli Arnarson BSc, PhD, (2019) *10 Types of Saturated Fats Reviewed,* on the Healthline website, <https://www.healthline.com/nutrition/saturated-fat-types>

Source 35 (Page 170) – A P Simopoulos; (2002), *The importance of the ratio of omega-6/omega-3 essential fatty acids,* the National Library of Medicine on the National Center for Biotechnology Information website, <https://pubmed.ncbi.nlm.nih.gov/12442909/>

Source 36 (Page 173) – Fred A Kummerow, (2009) *The negative effects of hydrogenated trans fats and what to do about them,* the National Library of Medicine on the National Center for Biotechnology Information website, <https://pubmed.ncbi.nlm.nih.gov/19345947/>

Source 37 (Page 178) – Canadian Sugar Institute, n.d., *Sources of Sugar,* on the Canadian Sugar Institute website, <https://sugar.ca/sugar-basics/sources-of-sugar>

Source 38 (Page 184) – Glycemic Index Research and GI News, n.d., *Everything you need to know about GI*, the Sydney University Glycemic Index Research Service (SUGiRS) on their website, <https://glycemicindex.com/>

Source 39 (Page 199) – The Sugar Association, n.d., *History of Sugar*, on The Sugar Association website, <https://www.sugar.org/sugar/history/>

Source 40 (Page 210) – Peter Howe, Jon Buckly and Barbara Meyer. (2007), *Long-chain omega-3 fatty acids in red meat*, on the Wiley.Online Library website, <https://onlinelibrary.wiley.com/doi/full/10.1111/j.1747-0080.2007.00201.x#>

Source 41 (Page 249) – *Eat a variety of healthy foods each day* Article published by Canada's Food Guide and published on the Government of Canada website

<https://food-guide.canada.ca/en/>

Source 42 (Page 255) – Anna-Britt Elisabet Agnsäter, <www.skbl.se/sv/artikel/AnnaBrittAgnsater>, Svenskt kvinnobiografiskt lexikon (article by Richard Tellström), retrieved 2024-01-25.

Source 43 (Page 256 & 262) – *Food Pyramids – What Should You Really Eat,* Downloadable Handout published by the Harvard T. H. Chan School of Public Health and available via their HSPH website:

<https://www.hsph.harvard.edu/wp-content/uploads/sites/30/2012/10/healthy-eating-pyramid-huds-handouts.pdf>

Downloads

There are downloadable copies of the various Food Tables, Planners and Diagrams which you can find at:

www.adietyoucanlivewith.com

They are available as Word Documents so you can adjust them if you prefer and print out at whatever paper size you prefer, A5, A4 etc.

You will also find a downloadable Word Doc with all the Online Sources with active links to speed things up if you want to check any of the articles, papers and other sources referred to throughout.

As you will be aware, the online links can change as websites are updated. Wherever possible I will keep the downloadable Word Doc as up to date as possible.

As I said right at the start, this book can never be finished, it is a work in progress so do feel free to re-visit the site to check for updates.

Cover Design

Cover designed by Getcovers. See: https://getcovers.com

Printed in Dunstable, United Kingdom

74903805R00163